Parenting a Dyslexic Child

Edited by
GILLIAN ASHLEY

FOREWORD BY GAVIN REID

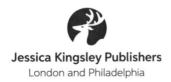

Jessica Kingsley Publishers
London and Philadelphia

First published in Great Britain in 2021 by Jessica Kingsley Publishers
An Hachette Company

1

Copyright © Jessica Kingsley Publishers 2021
Foreword copyright © Gavin Reid 2021

Front cover image source: Shutterstock®.

The fonts, layout and overall design of this book have been prepared
according to dyslexia-friendly principles. At JKP we aim to make our
books' content accessible to as many readers as possible.

All pages marked with a ★ can be downloaded at www.jkp.com/catalogue/
book/9781787754263 for personal use with this progamme, but may not be
reproduced for any other purposes without the permission of the publisher.

A CIP catalogue record for this title is available from the
British Library and the Library of Congress

ISBN 978 1 78775 426 3
eISBN 978 1 78775 427 0

Printed and bound in Great Britain by TJ Books Limited

Jessica Kingsley Publishers' policy is to use papers that are natural, renewable and recyclable
products and made from wood grown in sustainable forests. The logging and manufacturing
processes are expected to conform to the environmental regulations of the country of origin.

Jessica Kingsley Publishers
Carmelite House
50 Victoria Embankment
London EC4Y 0DZ

www.jkp.com

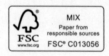

MIX
Paper from
responsible sources
FSC® C013056

Contents

Foreword

Parenting a Dyslexic Child is sure to be an essential book for all parents. Parents have been waiting for this type of book for many years and it is sure to be a massive hit!

Full of strategies and tips, written by accomplished and experienced authors, it covers all the essential areas from teaching strategies, assessment, supports, study skills and working with schools.

Parents need to have this book! It provides a comprehensive reference on dyslexia, a practical source of support and realistic pathways for progress. Parents often ask 'what should I do next?' – this book provides the answer in a comprehensive and clear manner. There are excellent chapters on the dyslexic brain, the identification and assessment process and practical ideas on supporting children with dyslexia from both professional and parent perspectives and also from an adult who has, and is experiencing dyslexia himself.

Gillian Ashley and the team of authors need to be congratulated in pulling together all the essential strands that can help ease the concerns of parents and provide them with a clear way forward and a bank of ideas and strategies that provides an understanding and a pathway to help them support their child.

This book will both inspire and inform. Essential reading for all parents with a child with dyslexia!

Gavin Reid

Introduction

This book is designed to give parents an overview of what dyslexia is, how it might affect your child, the assessment process and key transition points. The need for a handbook became apparent at the British Dyslexia Association as many parents shared their struggle engaging with a complicated education system as they try to understand why their child is having difficulties with reading and writing and fighting for support and a diagnosis.

Reading and writing are key skills which are required for accessing education, work and functions involved in everyday life. It is the importance of these skills and the fact that they are core skills needed for accessing learning in school which brings the enormity of a child's struggle to the forefront for parents. The book is designed to cover all of the pressing issues you might face as a family. Chapter 5 focuses on a full Diagnostic Assessment, what it is, who can assess, what is assessed and how the decision is made on whether it is dyslexia or not. Deciding whether to seek an assessment is one of the most important decisions you might make as a parent. For families who might decide not to have an assessment or might take time to decide, the book has many practical tips and strategies which will help you to work with your child in a multisensory way.

A quick road map of the book

In Chapter 1 the focus is on how the brain functions in tasks such as reading and spelling. There is a brief overview of which areas of the brain are involved in key cognitive skills, including working memory. The chapter explains some of the difficulties in finding a cause for dyslexia and how this has led to many definitions of dyslexia.

Chapter 2 includes a recap of some of the underlying cognitive difficulties associated with dyslexia and includes the Rose Report (2009) definition. The chapter highlights some of the emotional difficulties children and young people can experience and offers parents some concrete strategies for moving forwards.

Chapter 3 is written from a personal perspective and looks at strengths in dyslexia, as well as an exploration of assistive technology as a means of accessing reading and writing.

Chapter 4 focuses on the signs and indicators of dyslexia. In this chapter there are practical checklists, which are useful for parents as they provide a framework for thinking about some of the difficulties you may have already noticed. The checklists could be used as a starting point in trying to think about each indicator in relation to your child. These checklists are available to download from www.jkp.com/catalogue/book/9781787754263.

Chapter 5 is crucial reading if you are at the stage where you have decided to have your child assessed for dyslexia. This chapter takes you through what to expect, the differences between a Specialist Teacher and an Educational Psychologist, describes the different areas which are assessed and explains how a diagnosis is made.

Chapter 6 breaks down the specific difficulties of dyslexia

– reading, writing and spelling – and offers practical activities to address core skills. There are a lot of quick games and exercises you can practise with your child.

Organisational skills are a major stumbling point for many children and young people with dyslexia. Chapter 7 looks at organisational skills which might be impacted by issues with short-term memory. Having organisational difficulties can impact personal organisation, organisation of thoughts and organisation of time. The impact for a child is they might not have the right equipment, they might not plan their time effectively or they might struggle to collect their thoughts when working through written tasks. This chapter gives practical strategies for how you might help your child to develop strategies which enable more effective organisation.

Following on from organisational skills, Chapter 8 discusses study skills. Study skills is a term we tend to associate with study at a high level such as university, but learning and practising the skills involved are crucial for children with dyslexia. It is important they find strategies which work for them as we all extract and remember information differently. This chapter is practical and offers tips and strategies which you can begin to explore with your children from a young age.

As parents you are reliant on your child's school for help and advice, but crucially for the support they will put in place. Chapter 9 is important as it explores developing a positive dialogue with the school.

Finally, but most importantly, Chapter 10 covers self-esteem. If you are spending most of your time at school struggling to complete tasks, to keep up with your peers and to understand information, the cost of this is often lack of confidence and low self-esteem. This final chapter unpicks some of the difficult experiences your child might have had or be having. It also focuses on the development of self-esteem by looking for your child's strengths and ultimately developing them. It goes hand in hand that if we are doing things we are good at, we experience feeling successful. This chapter offers tips and strategies on how to build these experiences, which can then impact on how your child feels.

Many of the enquiries which are received at the British Dyslexia Association are for practical information about how to find an assessor or what parents can ask the school to provide. However, mostly, parents will share their experience, frustrations and how helpless they feel. This handbook is intended to provide answers to many questions for parents in one book.

In conclusion, I hope you find the book useful and it enables you to navigate your child's learning journey successfully.

Gillian Ashley

Reference

Rose, J. (2009) *Identifying and Teaching Children and Young People with Dyslexia and Literacy Difficulties*. Nottingham: DCSF.

CHAPTER 1

The Dyslexic Brain

GILLIAN ASHLEY

Summary

- Dyslexia, definitions and underlying causes.

- Reading and the brain.

- Brain scans.

- Working memory and the brain.

Dyslexia is a specific learning difficulty (SpLD) which affects the ability to read, spell and write. It is one of several conditions which come under the umbrella term specific learning difficulties. Dyslexia is specific because the challenges associated with it affect the skills involved in reading and spelling. Dyslexia affects our access to written language, which is a crucial form of communication. Before we acquire access to a written language we learn to speak as a key means of communicating. We move through a variety of stages from babbling to naming animals to saying key words and on to sentences. The development of our vocabulary is reinforced through our families and they are instrumental in modelling language at an early stage.

Examples of other conditions that fall within the term specific learning difficulties include:

- dyspraxia

- attention deficit hyperactivity disorder (ADHD)

- dyscalculia

- autism

- speech and language delay.

Specific learning difficulties commonly co-occur and there are aspects such as working memory difficulties which are associated with several conditions.

As we enter school, learning to read is another means we have of communicating and gaining knowledge. It is the core business of primary schools to teach reading and writing. Equally, it is the expectation of parents that their children will learn to read and write in school. Schools use a system of teaching reading which is called synthetic phonics. This involves matching a sound with a letter, out to letter strings which are blended to make a word. For many parents the first sign of a difficulty might be with basic recognition of a letter and being able to say the sound. As this is taught in schools, it is when children attend school that parents might first notice a difficulty. For many children it is the first time they begin to work through the stages of learning to read. It is also the beginning of a journey of failure for children with dyslexia as they struggle to break through the code involved in reading and spelling.

If we think of our own learning journeys, we will be able to identify aspects of school which we found easy and some we found difficult. We might have gravitated to areas of the curriculum which sparked our interest more and as adults we might be able to link this to the careers we have gone on to have.

One of the keys to the road map through education is to understand what the strengths and weaknesses are for your child. Enabling children to feel successful in some areas of the curriculum might balance the lack of confidence and feelings of failure in other areas.

The recognition that reading is a difficult skill to learn is not new. In the late 1960s, Goodman (1967) referred to reading as a 'psycholinguistic guessing game'. This accurately reflects the experience children have when they try to crack the code to access text. For many children guessing is their main strategy and is mostly based on the visual shape of the word. It is unlikely the word they guess will have the same or similar meaning and this contributes to children failing to gain any meaning from what they have attempted to read. Trying again to read the same passage a child has struggled to read does not give them access to text and it is this repeated cycle which can be hard to break. Many dyslexia specialists might refer to these difficulties as being at the behavioural level as reading and spelling are the outward behaviour of processes which are cognitive and brain related.

There are three levels of processes:

◇ The brain level: anything brain related (when reading and writing) is found or could be placed here.

◇ The cognitive level: the phonological processing involved in reading and writing.

◇ The behavioural level: reading and writing.

Specialists may locate a point of breakdown in the reading and writing processes. They can then design an evidence-based intervention that addresses the breakdown points.

Despite a wealth of research into the cause of dyslexia, it can be confusing for parents to generally understand as there is a variety of definitions and a lack of consensus on what causes dyslexia. Although there is no single agreed definition of dyslexia, there are common elements in the definitions. Most agree that it is a language-based difficulty which is neurobiological in basis. It affects reading, spelling and writing, which can be explained by difficulties with working memory, visual and verbal processing or phonological processing.[1] Some definitions state that it is a life-long condition.

Many parents ask why we have not been able to definitely say what causes dyslexia when we have access to brain scans and other types of technology. Answering this question is

---

1   Working memory is the part of the memory we use when we undertake complex cognitive tasks such as driving and following directions or writing and listening at the same time. The tasks are usually goal oriented. We are doing them for a purpose or outcome. Phonological processing describes how we use sounds to access and to process both spoken and written language. For instance, when we are stuck on a word when reading we might break the work into individual sounds which we then blend to help us to read the word.

not so simple. This is because the research area is wide and varied; for example, some research focuses on eye tracking when we read, whilst others have looked at how the working memory affects reading and spelling. Each individual piece of research does not necessarily seek to find out what the cause is; instead the focus is on specific elements which might explain a difficulty associated with dyslexia.

The most well known of the theories is that the initial underlying cause is a phonological deficit. The phonological deficit explores the difficulties in the reading process and explains this as an impairment in the way the brain represents spoken language. This causal theory acknowledges there are difficulties wider than reading which people with dyslexia experience. Other common theories are the Cerebellum, the Magnocellular and the Double Deficit. The Cerebellum supports some of the phonological deficit as it asserts the issue is an abnormality in the brain. The theory identifies issues with motor control, balance, working memory, attention and automatisation. Some of the areas are associated with reading, for example working memory and automatisation. The Magnocelluar theory attempts to bring together the causes by showing there is a dysfunction in the visual, auditory and tactile pathways of the magnocellular system.

The Double Deficit theory pinpoints two aspects, rapid naming and phonological impairments. It emphasises the importance of being able to match a sound to a letter but this needs to be done quickly.

Each theory has explored different aspects, but all include an explanation at the brain level. Brain scanning has enabled an in-depth analysis of the functions of the brain when carrying out different skills. This has led to a range of discoveries made from speech production to interactions within the language parts of the brain and motor automaticity. Motor automaticity is the fluency between the brain's instructions to the action. The action could be speaking. We do not have to give this any attention as it is an automatic skill for most of us. Another barrier to identifying a single cause is how complex the brain is. It is not fully understood how the different areas of the brain interact to enable us to carry out all of the many functions we undertake as humans.

Some facts about the brain:

- The brain consists of 100 billion neurons.

- Neurons are messengers which send and receive information between different areas of the brain and the senses, making them critical in the learning process.

- The brain is made up of approximately 75 per cent water. Dehydration of the brain can impair memory and performance.

- An adult brain weighs 1.36kg (3lb).

The brain is the organ in the body which enables us to think, plan, learn, make decisions and access language. When we are reading we are engaging perceptual and cognitive processes as we need to do things like visually perceive letter shapes and decide which letter it is and which sound it represents. Access to a wide vocabulary is essential as it enables our understanding of what we have read. Spelling is viewed as harder to master as the English language has what is known as a deep orthography. This means the rules of spelling are not straightforward, as different combinations of letters can represent the same sound. Take the word 'rain' as an example. The difficult sound is the long 'a'. There are several ways of writing the long 'a' sound and this might cause confusion for dyslexic people who are not sure which long 'a' is correct (e.g. rain, rane, rein, ran, raen).

In primary school reading is taught using a synthetic phonics approach, which encourages children to learn the sound associated with each letter. They will be taught phonological awareness skills such as blending sounds to make a word and segmenting words into sounds. These skills involve an area of the brain called the temporal lobe. The temporal lobe also enables us to discriminate between sounds. This is important when we are learning the different sounds associated with letters as they can often look and sound similar, for example M and N. Verbal memory is also used in this process. Being able to hold a letter string in the memory is essential before blending. Verbal memory is found in the temporal lobe. Confusion in differentiating between the sounds could indicate a hearing difficulty, an auditory processing difficulty or a gap in learning. A difficulty connected to the visual elements in reading could be as a result of issues with sight. It is important for schools and families to consider and eliminate any other reason why there might be a difficulty before undertaking a dyslexia assessment.

Once we have put sounds together to make a word, saying the word, whether in our mind or out loud, involves the Broca's area in the brain. Understanding of what we have read is also located here. The Broca's area is situated in the frontal lobe. There are several brain areas which are involved with language and they each have a specific job, but they also interact with each other as we undertake some of the skills involved in reading.

As well as an auditory element, in order for us to begin any decoding of written words for reading, we have to look at the words first. We have to identify the letters and understand and process what the brain sees using visual perception (visual processing) skills. Visual perception is found in the occiptal lobe in the brain. Research in this area has more recently focused on eye movements, through tracking what happens visually. We might think when reading our eyes move smoothly across the text, but in fact, they move in quick jerks called saccades. Between the saccades are fixations. Some research has looked at the amount of words/text which contains useful information and which can be obtained on each fixation (Rayner *et al.* 2012). What they found is we fixate on 80 per cent of content words such as nouns and 20 per cent of function words such as the, or, a. This means we are more likely to omit function words when reading as they are easily processed.

You might have noticed when listening to your own child that they miss out small words. If meaning is maintained even though the words are omitted it will not affect the overall comprehension. We do not have to be 100 per cent accurate when reading to extract meaning and have a good, meaningful experience. Errors in reading are important to note as they can explain where a point of breakdown is, for example, if substitution is a common error, it could suggest a lack of decoding strategies; whereas a reliance on sounding each letter could point to difficulties with blending or an overload in memory.

To bring all of this together, when we read and spell we are accessing different parts of the brain. These different parts light up when they are active in the reading process. Brain scans have enabled us to understand which areas light up when undertaking different skills involved in reading. A difficulty in learning to read could indicate a breakdown in one of these processes, such as phonological awareness or verbal memory. The key to success in reading and spelling is being able to pinpoint where the breakdown is. The problem is we do not have access to brain scans at home or in a classroom setting and this is where observations are crucial in identifying what children do or do not do when they read and write.

Brain scans have enabled us to discover which parts of the brain we are accessing when reading and spelling. The most common scans used are:

- **Event related potentials (ERP)**: This type of scan monitors the pattern of electrical brain activity. It enables us to understand the timing of a variety of cognitive processes precisely.

- **Functional Magnetic Resonance Imaging (fMRI)**: This scan shows an image of the blood oxygenation and it gives us information about the location of an event and timing involved.

- **Positron Emission Tomography (PET)**: Neural activity is measured using this scan.

The main point to remember with any cognitive task we perform is that the brain will play a huge part in the process. We cannot exclude from this chapter the working memory. The memory, simply put, enables us to remember information. How does the brain store information? We process so much information during the course of a day, we could not possibly remember it all, nor would we want to, as some information is not useful for us in the long term. When we receive a piece of information we hold it for seconds in our short-term memory; this can be auditory or visual. At this point we can forget the information, use it or store it. Most of the tasks we ask children to complete in school or college involve the working memory. This is where we are manipulating the information. This sounds complex and it is.

Imagine you are watching a very interesting programme and you decide to make some notes whilst you listen. You are accessing your working memory as you are listening and picking out the main points which you write down in notes. Children might find when they are free-writing a sentence, they hold this in their memory whilst they write. If they get stuck on a spelling they are then going through the process of working out which letters they are writing whilst holding their sentence in their memory.

The working memory is a core part of our higher order thinking like planning. Planning and organisation difficulties are often associated with dyslexia. When we think about the working memory, it is clear that it is critical to all of the learning tasks we undertake. We could go a step further and say it is critical to pretty much everything the brain does. Like most of our understanding about the brain, it is not fully understood how the working memory works. Like our understanding of dyslexia, there is not an agreed consensus on the complexities of the working memory. This is an area where there is a lot of research being undertaken to enable us to better understand the process.

The brain and dyslexia are huge things to understand. We have not got a simple explanation of dyslexia, nor are we sure which parts of the brain are responsible for each part involved in the process of reading. The important message for you as a parent is that research into how the brain works is extensive and ongoing, and research findings are enabling us to make better sense of what we are observing in our children. Our observations of individual children enable us to plan programmes which suit each child's particular spread of difficulties.

🔖 Key takeaways

- Dyslexia is a specific learning difficulty which affects the skills involved in reading, writing and spelling.

- Difficulties with phonological awareness, verbal memory and verbal processing speed are characteristic features associated with dyslexia.

- The skills involved in reading and spelling all engage different parts of the brain.

- Working memory difficulties are commonly associated with dyslexia.

- Working memory is critical to all learning tasks.

References

Goodman, K. (1967) 'Reading: A psycholinguistic guessing game.' *Journal of the Reading Specialist 6*, 4, 126–135.

Rayner, K., Pollatsek, A., Ashby, J. & Clifton, C.J. (2012) *Psychology of Reading* (2nd ed.). New York, London: Psychology Press.

CHAPTER 2

Overview of Dyslexia and Support Strategies

DR LINDSAY PEER CBE

Summary

- ◇ What is dyslexia?

- ◇ Ways dyslexia can impact a child.

- ◇ Behavioural and emotional challenges for dyslexic children and their families.

- ◇ What you can do to support your child.

- ◇ Where to go for professional support.

'I just can't do it... Don't tell me I should know, or say I'm not listening or trying hard enough because I am... I must be stupid! My brain doesn't work properly!'

Parents and carers across the world have heard these heartbreaking and distressing cries from their dyslexic youngsters. They have witnessed books thrown across the room, pencils being broken, and homework and schoolbooks torn up – often followed by floods of tears.

The following comments have been made to me by children and young people with regards to their challenges at school:

◇ 'I must be an idiot.'

◇ 'I can't read/spell/remember my times tables/learn French. They say I have to work harder but I'm trying as hard as I can, and I just can't do it.'

◇ 'My younger sister can read better than me; that upsets me.'

◇ 'They speak too fast; I just don't get it.'

◇ 'People know less than me but get better marks, just because teachers can't read my writing. I can't get my ideas on paper and that's all that matters to them... It's not fair.'

◇ 'I'm a failure... I have no future.'

There is an ongoing struggle to keep up with the pace of their class. They find it hard to commit their well-formed ideas to paper, and often underachieve in written tests even when they understand and know the subject matter. For some, although they can discuss the subject matter in class, they cannot remember it afterwards.

As a consequence of the ongoing daily struggles, emotional issues often occur – including stress, anxiety, frustration, low self-esteem, demotivation, lack of confidence and depression. This then impacts upon the entire family. It is all so very hard for everyone concerned – the youngster, parents, siblings and school staff.

The sadness for me is that there is still insufficient understanding that dyslexic youngsters can be able, even very able, and with the right input would reach their potential academically and feel better about themselves.

I'm asked the same types of questions from parents and carers all over the world. They include:

◇ What is dyslexia? Is it an illness?

◇ If you are diagnosed dyslexic as a child, will you always be dyslexic?

◇ Are all children who can't read well dyslexic? Can you be dyslexic if you can read?

◇ Do all dyslexic people reverse letters, words and symbols when writing?

◇ Homework is such a battle. What should we do?

◇ Why does my child do okay in spelling tests, after we've gone over and over them, but still can't remember those words when writing an essay? They will sometimes even write the same word in three different ways in one piece of work.

◇ If I'm dyslexic, will my child be?

◇ I have other children who have dyspraxia, dyscalculia or attention difficulties. Are these things related?

◇ Why isn't my child's teacher trained to teach dyslexic children?

◇ What can I do to help?

◇ How can I help my youngster believe in themselves?

◇ Will they be able to secure and hold down a job which matches their ability and interests?

There are many reasons why youngsters struggle with reading and not all of those youngsters will be dyslexic. Some may not have had access to books and show little interest in the written word as they get older. They may not know the language of instruction. They might say they find reading boring and want to play electronic games instead. They may perhaps have other difficulties. They will need specific and targeted help depending upon their needs to help them engage and reach their potential.

The KPMG report *The Long Term Costs of Literacy Difficulties* (KPMG Foundation 2006), found that:

◇ the largest group of people with SEN are those with literacy difficulties

◇ there is a link to anti-social behaviour

◇ there is a greater risk of truancy and exclusion

◇ such learners were ultimately less likely to take public examinations

◇ a large number of boys felt that school was a waste of time

◇ those with English as an additional language (EAL) were often overlooked

◇ people with literacy difficulties were less likely to be employed, and if at work, were likely to be in jobs which were lower paid

⬧ their own children had lower reading scores

⬧ there was a greater chance of homelessness and/or criminality.

These negatives must be avoided at all costs. But, with early identification, understanding, empathy and appropriate skilled teaching, these children have every hope for the future and considerable opportunities for success.

So, what is dyslexia? The most commonly used description of dyslexia is from the 2009 Rose Report (a significant review of UK support for young people with dyslexia and literacy difficulties):

⬧ Dyslexia is a learning difficulty that primarily affects the skills involved in accurate and fluent word reading and spelling.

⬧ Characteristic features of dyslexia are difficulties in phonological awareness, verbal memory and verbal processing speed.

⬧ Dyslexia occurs across the range of intellectual abilities.

⬧ It is best thought of as a continuum, not a distinct category, and there are no clear cut-off points.

⬧ Co-occurring difficulties may be seen in aspects of language, motor coordination, mental calculation, concentration and personal organisation, but these are not, by themselves, markers of dyslexia.

⬧ A good indication of the severity and persistence of dyslexic difficulties can be gained by examining how the individual responds or has responded to well-founded intervention.

In addition to these characteristics, the British Dyslexia Association (2009) further acknowledges the visual and auditory processing difficulties that some individuals with dyslexia can experience and points out that dyslexic readers can show a combination of abilities and difficulties that affect the learning process. Some also have strengths in other areas, such as design, problem solving, creative skills, interactive skills and oral skills.

Many dyslexic children are identified through their failure to acquire effective literacy skills and their struggle at school. If we look into their histories, many of these children experienced early difficulties with aspects of language skills; this is not surprising as dyslexia is a language-based difficulty. Parents often report early developmental challenges in areas such as the acquisition of phonics, glue ear, auditory processing and working memory.

Overlap with other specific learning differences

We need to note too that there is a considerable overlap with other specific learning difficulties such as dyscalculia, dyspraxia and attention deficit disorder, as well as auditory processing. It is not unusual for dyslexic youngsters to have more than one condition, although that is not always the case.

Sometimes a child might have one or more of the conditions, and a sibling may have a different one. We cannot put all dyslexic children in one basket; they are all different, with their unique set of strengths and challenges and levels of resilience.

Working memory

Memory weakness at school is something that sometimes surprises parents. A youngster may be able to remember a film they have seen or a holiday they enjoyed the year before without difficulty, but have problems retaining learning.

There are indeed different types of memory. Dyslexic youngsters tend to have fewer difficulties with long-term memory but more with working memory. In the classroom, problems tend to be seen in areas like times tables, spelling, historical dates, formulae, and reworking and processing visual and auditory information.

Listening challenges

Listening is essential at school, and youngsters who experience difficulties in this area will struggle. In young children, such difficulties can sometimes be confused with hearing loss and/or auditory processing difficulties.

Hearing loss prevents sound reaching the auditory nervous system.

Youngsters with auditory processing difficulties/disorder (APD), however, often have hearing levels that are within the normal range, or sometimes hypersensitive. APD is more of a listening problem, likely sited on the auditory neural pathways. It is thought that up to 70 per cent of dyslexic children have APD.[1]

Both lead to challenges listening, particularly in noisy backgrounds. This also has the potential to affect language development in the young, and social interaction.

Filling in missing auditory information is an emergent skill.

---

1 See www.auditorycenter.com/what-is-auditory-processing-disorder/ prevalence-of-apd.

Pauline Grant, Teacher of the Deaf and Lead Consultant at *Listen to Learn*, interestingly notes that only by approximately 15 years of age are higher-level language and auditory skills fully developed.[2] Therefore, when we ask children to listen, we must not expect them to respond as adults might. We must adjust our expectations.[3]

To learn more about glue ear and the overlap with dyslexia, see the book *Glue Ear* by Lindsay Peer (2005).

For those with APD type difficulties/disorder, treat as you might for those with hearing loss, for example, they may need an FM radio hearing aid and wireless receiver. Reduce background noise by acoustically treating the room(s) and ensure good lip-reading conditions. Switch off low level humming (e.g. radiators and computers) where possible. Always gain the attention of the youngster before speaking to them by first saying their name and facing them. Speak clearly and slightly louder than normal but do not exaggerate your speech. Be careful not to speak whilst your back is to them.

Visual challenges

Some dyslexic youngsters have difficulties visually following the written word. They may, for example, perceive letters to be moving around or blurred, experience tracking difficulties, switch letters and/or symbols around, perceive the white between the words, and need to reread for information.

---

2   Personal communication.
3   See BSA APD Practice Guidance (2018) for further information, www.thebsa.org.uk/wp-content/uploads/2018/02/Position-Statement-and-Practice-Guidance-APD-2018.pdf.

Speed, accuracy and comprehension are likely to be affected as well as the ability to remember.[4]

Not all dyslexic youngsters have these visual challenges and some can indeed read sufficiently well whilst experiencing other difficulties mentioned.

For those with visual difficulties related to the written word, if an assessment is not possible, then speak to teachers about trying the following strategies:

- ◇ Check the size and font. Personally, I prefer 12 point, 1.5 spacing in Verdana; others might like Ariel. Whatever suits the youngster best, I suggest you use.

- ◇ Ask if they cannot read certain colours on the board.

- ◇ Change the background colour on the electronic whiteboard and their personal screens. An off-white colour is likely to help others too.

- ◇ Coloured notebooks may help some.

- ◇ Use a tracking line.

- ◇ Use a Reader Pen.

- ◇ Write in alternate line colours when writing on board.

- ◇ Leave space in worksheets – easier access.

- ◇ Use the technique SQ4R (survey, question, read, recite, review, relate).

- ◇ Enlarge worksheets and examination papers if appropriate.

---

4   See www.babo.co.uk for further information.

◇ To encourage reluctant readers, look at the Barrington Stoke books, which are designed with the dyslexic youngster in mind. There are also worksheets to use with them.

Literacy development

The Literacy Trust (2017) defines literacy as 'the ability to read, write, speak and listen in a way that lets us communicate effectively and make sense of the world'. For effective understanding of the written word, we need reasonably good listening comprehension and decoding skills; to be able to read automatically allows greater space for understanding. Work gets harder and demands become faster paced as we get older, and the lack of effective underlying learning skills and literacy skills greatly affects success across the curriculum.

For younger children, phonological methods which are structured, sequential and multisensory are useful. Programmes such as *Alpha to Omega* by Prof. Beve Hornsby and *Read Write Inc.* by Ruth Miskin are commonly used programmes for dyslexic children.[5] Use them as set out so that they reinforce learning. Jumping around within the books is not appropriate.

When slightly older, if a phonological method has not worked, then a meaning based morphological approach might be useful. (This approach considers how words are formed, and their relationship to other words in the same language.) This will bypass the challenges for youngsters

---

5   See https://www.pearsonschoolsandfecolleges.co.uk/secondary/English AndMedia/11-14/AlphaToOmega/AlphaToOmega.aspx and https://www. ruthmiskin.com/en/find-out-more/parents for further information.

with poor phonological skills. See *Red Hot Root Words* Books 1 and 2 by Dianne Draze (2005a, 2005b).

For those who experience difficulties with handwriting, there are a number of programmes available to help – occupational therapists are sometimes also asked to advise. If writing is illegible, if there is pain in the hand when writing or production of work is far too slow, then typing might be considered. There are a number of touch-typing programmes available, including *Nessy Fingers* for younger children, *Touch-type Read and Spell* and *Typing Instructor for Kids* by Helen Arkell, all of which also help reinforce spelling.

Behavioural and emotional considerations

Time is the greatest gift to give any child with special educational needs. Dyslexia can be managed well. Try to rid yourself of any self-doubt as a parent and find support groups to help you learn how to manage the highs and the lows, the frustrations and the upsets as well as the fears. Remember that you know your child better than anyone, and whilst teachers are rightly responsible for whole classes, you have only your child to think about and you are the expert for your child.

The *most* important thing of all is to believe in your child and to do the best you can to show them that you do. Ignore comments such as, 'Well, you would say that wouldn't you because you're my Mum/Dad.' Show them their successes – ideally in a visual, perhaps graphic, way.

◇ Listen to them with real focus. Don't tell them that what they are saying isn't right, as it is their perception and it is true for them. Try seeing things through their eyes. Remember that if the problem is school-related, they have to be there for many, many hours a day, a week, a year. If you were really unhappy at your job, you might try and move, and perhaps move again until it feels right. Our children have to go to school; they do not have many alternative options.

◇ Accept them for who they are and tell them how you will try and help them find ways to get on better and feel better.

◇ Point out that dyslexia is a combination of strengths as well as challenges. Focus upon strengths and interests too, so that they become as good as they can in at least one area.

◇ Try and find a way to work together by asking for help from school, family members and friends. The British Dyslexia Association also has local Dyslexia Associations across the country. Perhaps join your nearest one and find other families in the same position. There you will learn more about dyslexia, overlapping conditions, self-advocacy, and your youngster's rights, thereby empowering yourself. You can find out where the best places are to go for local help, schools that may have more specialism – and be able to introduce your youngster to others like themselves.

◇ If they can meet those with dyslexia who have done well in the local area, this might help as they could be good role models. Find ways to speak to successful dyslexic people you know and hear their stories. This may help by reinforcing the positive and showing them that they can overcome hurdles with persistence.

◇ You may have a Dyslexia Friendly School in your area, which is helpful for those with milder needs. If more severe, then specialist teaching may well become necessary.

Some emotional messages to get across to your youngster are that they should:

◇ find their areas of interest and work towards achieving those goals; nobody should stop them

◇ find the people who have the skills to help and then work with them

◇ be as focused and determined as possible

◇ learn from their mistakes – a great strategy

◇ remember that they are unique; they have strengths that others do not have – work with those strengths

◇ believe in themselves

◇ realise that computers offer great opportunities; become as proficient as possible with them

◇ remember that they can only make a dream come true if they have a dream.

Getting support for your dyslexic child

Share your concerns with school, specifically class teachers and the SENCO (Special Educational Needs Co-ordinator). Aim for the ideal – the voice of the youngster is heard, and that school and home all work together with them. Discuss with school how homework is to be managed and see the book *Taking the Hell Out of Homework* by Neil MacKay (2011) for helpful ideas. Ensure that the youngster is never kept in at breaktime to complete work as they need their rest or a chance to run around even more than others.

It may become the case, when all regular avenues are exhausted, that a request for the support of the Local Authority's Educational Psychologist is made. If that is not possible, you may wish to find an independent professional. Likewise, it may be helpful to get an assessment from a speech and language therapist, occupational therapist, and if there are mental health issues, either Child and Adolescent Mental Health Services (CAMHS) or an independent psychiatrist or psychologist. In some cases, needs are so great that an Education, Health and Care Plan (EHCP) is warranted to support and protect your child.

With understanding, support and appropriate teaching, dyslexic children have the potential to do well and achieve in life. Never give up!

℘ Key takeaways

- Dyslexia is a language-based difficulty leading to differences in learning.

- Very many dyslexic people have strengths alongside challenges.

- Underlying difficulties include working memory, processing of auditory and/or visual information and phonological skills.

- Failure and ongoing difficulties may lead to emotional challenges.

- Dyslexia can commonly co-occur with other specific learning differences, such as dyspraxia, dyscalculia and attention deficit disorder.

- There are many things you can do at home to support your dyslexic child.

- There are many experts that can help your child with their dyslexia; sometimes these can be accessed free through your child's school.

References

British Dyslexia Association (2009) 'What is dyslexia?' Accessed on November 28, 2020 at https://www.bdadyslexia.org.uk/dyslexia/about-dyslexia/what-is-dyslexia.

Draze, D. (2005a) *Red Hot Root Words Book 1: Mastering Vocabulary with Prefixes, Suffixes and Root Words*. Waco, TX: Prufrock Press.

Draze, D. (2005b) *Red Hot Root Words Book 2: Mastering Vocabulary with Prefixes, Suffixes and Root Words*. Waco, TX: Prufrock Press.

KPMG Foundation (2006) *The Long Term Costs of Literacy Difficulties*. London: KPMG Foundation.

Literacy Trust, The (2017) 'What is literacy?' Accessed on October 26, 2020 at https://literacytrust.org.uk/information/what-is-literacy.

MacKay, N. (2011) *Taking the Hell Out of Homework: Tips and Techniques for Parents and Home Educators*. Wakefield: SEN Marketing.

Peer, L. (2005) *Glue Ear: An Essential Guide for Teachers, Parents and Health Professionals*. Abingdon: Routledge.

Rose, J. (2009) *Identifying and Teaching Children and Young People with Dyslexia and Literacy Difficulties*. Nottingham: DCSF.

Further reading

Braaten, E. & Willoughby, B. (2014) *Bright Kids Who Can't Keep Up: Help Your Child Overcome Slow Processing Speed and Succeed in a Fast-Paced World*. New York, London: Guilford Press.

Chivers, M.L. (2019) *Alli Can't Write: A Storybook for Children with Handwriting Difficulties Including those with: Dyslexia, Dysgraphia, Dyscalculia, Dyspraxia & ADHD*. UK: M.L. Chivers.

Cooper-Kahn, J. & Dietzel, L.C. (2008) *Late, Lost, and Unprepared: A Parents' Guide to Helping Children with Executive Functioning*. Bethesda, MD: Woodbine House.

Mountjoy, A. (2018) *Can I Tell You About Auditory Processing Disorder?* London: Jessica Kingsley Publishers.

Peer, L. & Reid, G. (eds) (2020) *Special Educational Needs: A Guide for Inclusive Practice* (3rd ed.). Los Angeles, CA: SAGE.

CHAPTER 3

Dyslexia Top Tips from the Perspective of Someone with Dyslexia

ADAM GORDON

Summary

- ◇ Dyslexia is different in every individual.

- ◇ The importance of focusing on strengths.

- ◇ How role models can build confidence.

- ◇ Why dyslexia shouldn't stop a love of reading and writing.

- ◇ How coping strategies and assistive technology can help.

My first school didn't work out. I don't remember exactly how it went, but I believe it was politely suggested that I'd be better off somewhere else! Over the next year or two I was in a terrible 'special school' and was eventually diagnosed with dyslexia. I then moved into a specialist dyslexia school – and that was the start of things really changing for the better for me and my relationship with education.

I later went to a specialist dyslexia secondary school, achieved GCSEs, an A Level, GNVQ and ultimately completed a degree. None of these things would have happened without the support I received from my family and amazing teachers.

Since then, I've had quite a few different jobs but what has brought me to contributing this chapter is my most recent history.

Over the past 13 years I have been working in special educational needs settings. Initially I was a teaching assistant, then a teacher, assistant headteacher, school leader and now, having left teaching, I hold a senior position in the educational technology sector working for a charitable trust called LGfL. My role centres on special educational needs, inclusion and wellbeing.

I've learned many lessons through my own journey and continue to do so. I think that there are some lessons I was aware of at the time and some that I identified in hindsight. I will now expand on the top tips mentioned in the chapter title.

Top tip one: Understanding

Everyone supporting a child with dyslexia should seek to really understand *all* their strengths and areas of challenge. This includes family, school staff and, most of all, the young person themselves.

Managing self-esteem and resilience is incredibly important. I have never seen my dyslexia as a disability. I see it as a difference and I've always felt that different can be good.

The various ways in which my dyslexia impacts upon me

can certainly present challenges. It should be noted that those challenges will vary from one dyslexic person to another.

What is much more disabling is having low resilience and low self-esteem. We live at a time where, in the UK at least, people are finally waking up to the vital importance of good mental health for all of us. Every person will have their own specific challenges, but I believe that many dyslexic young people are at high risk, and the following quote sums up why:

> Everybody's a genius. But if you judge a fish by its ability to climb a tree, it will spend its whole life believing that it is stupid. (Author unknown, but commonly attributed to Albert Einstein)

Our education system has evolved over decades to meet the needs of society at a point in time. However, society and the workplace have changed beyond recognition, whilst schools really have not. Therefore, many ways of teaching and, in fact, skills being taught play to the challenges of dyslexia rather than harnessing the strengths of each individual. This can be hugely stressful and make dyslexic people feel they aren't good enough or are indeed 'stupid'.

When we understand what these challenges are, we can put in place incredibly simple support that may well change people's experience of education and ultimately the course of their lives.

Top tip two: Focus on strengths

Build on the individual's strengths and interests. It can help shore up their self-esteem and resilience when they are finding other stuff difficult. It can help turn, 'I'm stupid and worthless' into, 'This thing is difficult right now'.

Many dyslexic learners (like most people) have interests and talents in which they excel. It can be the case that their ability to think differently will give them a competitive edge, notably in areas such as sport, design and art. Unfortunately, these areas of strength are not near the top of the hierarchy of subjects in our education system. This can mean they are not celebrated and encouraged – despite the fact they may well lead to successful career paths.

Top tip three: Find role models

Role models can help raise young people's aspirations and show that dyslexia is not going to be the thing that stops them succeeding. There are hundreds of famous examples, but a role model could just as easily be a teacher or family member.

The benefit of seeing that 'someone who is like me' has been successful cannot be underestimated. There are huge numbers of well-known personalities across every field from science to acting and from literature to sports who, by their example, prove that dyslexia need not stop you being ambitious about your future. But not all role models have to be famous. Just do an internet search: you and your young person will be surprised by the names and fields of many dyslexic high achievers.

A family member, friend of the family, teacher or possibly you yourself can demonstrate that although dyslexia might make some things a bit more difficult, that's not the end of the story – these challenges can be overcome.

Top tip four: Dyslexia doesn't mean you can't love language

Don't let dyslexia ruin a love of reading and writing.

I love language. I always have.

My writing is okay, but I am lucky that I get help with editing my work from an incredibly patient colleague when something is for public consumption. For things that aren't directly related to my day job, such as this chapter, I've got wonderful friends and family who will look over it before you get to read it. Often, there is not that much to do because I run it through incredibly powerful technology before sending it out to others to read. If your ears pricked up at my first mention of technology, then be patient, more information is coming up soon (see my fifth top tip).

I was able to read individual words well most of the way through school, but this will get you only so far. It makes reading a laborious and utilitarian task.

When I was about 15, we were on a family holiday and I picked up one of my dad's spy novels that he'd finished with. I started reading and *boom*! I saw the story unfolding in my mind. I'd finally got to a level of fluency and found the right book about a topic I enjoyed, and I haven't looked back. I still read very slowly but well enough to get what reading is all about. I've been fascinated, thrilled and enthralled by what I have read.

Audiobooks existed in my childhood but were not as readily available as they are now. Scanners and text to speech technology were in their infancy and not available to most people. Things are different now and we'll go into this in more detail in my fifth top tip.

For me what sustained my love of stories and made me want to be able to read them for myself was my sister. She has been an insatiable bookworm for as long as I can remember. She was also incredibly patient and kind, in that rather than just reading to herself at night (which I'm sure would have been more enjoyable) she read out loud. I would sit or lie on her bedroom floor and listen and really get into the stories. Not everyone has an Emma. But luckily, these days you don't need an Emma, you might have an Alexa instead!

Some people just don't love stories and literature, but please, please make sure that dyslexia is not the reason for this.

Earlier, I talked about working to strengths. There is no universal statement you can make about dyslexic people as we are all different, but bear in mind that many dyslexic people are phenomenal verbal communicators. Never forget that writing is not the only important use of language.

Top tip five: Find coping strategies that work for the individual

It's difficult to talk in too much detail about general day-to-day strategies as these can be so wide ranging and are usually something that people will develop for themselves (sometimes with support).

My dyslexia means my working memory is absolutely appalling. As a kid I used to lose stuff all the time. About ten years ago a flatmate pointed out to me that I patted myself down every time we left the house. I thought about it a bit and realised that every time I leave work or home, I subconsciously touch my own pockets to check I have my wallet, travel card, phone and keys – and what's more, there is never any variation, each of these items goes in the same place every single day. I really don't think about it but if I touch my back-left pocket and my wallet isn't there, I'll notice and make sure I get it. Having a routine or just getting a consistent habit can be helpful. So, whether it's conscious or it happens automatically, really trying to build some habits to help avoid mistakes can be useful.

Technology has evolved and continues to develop and plays to the strengths of many dyslexic people. I was taught to touch type at school, and it's been an incredibly powerful tool that has opened opportunities to me that would not have existed otherwise. If I was ten years older, I'm not sure I'd have managed university as I don't think I could have got through using pencil and paper. Even a typewriter would have made things extremely difficult.

There is so much to cover here. In the following list, I am aiming to keep to mainstream technology that is either free or included in devices and software most people have access to at home or at school.

⬦ Spell and grammar check is commonplace and used by so many people that we take it for granted. These tools are increasing in power with the rise of artificial intelligence; they can improve writing in a range of ways.

⬦ Touch typing, as mentioned above, is an invaluable skill if you can take the time to learn to do it well.

⬦ There is an incredible number of technologies out there that will read the written and typed word for you (called text to speech software). Apple, Google and Microsoft hardware and software all have this capability. There are also lots of free apps and browser extensions that can support in this way. I often use text to speech to proofread my emails before sending them. I'd like to say I do it before I send every email, but the truth is, I tend to remember to do it for big important emails or emails to new people who don't know me. I pick up virtually all of my mistakes this way. When I read it back to myself, I miss most of my own mistakes. I'm not sure why exactly but I just can't proofread my own work.

◇ Capabilities are commonly built in that will convert what you're saying into written words (known as speech to text). They perform very well and cost you nothing with no set up required in most cases. This can be used to get ideas down without any need for writing or typing. I type very well, and my spelling isn't terrible these days. However, if I come to a word that I'm stuck with and I can't get close enough for my spell checker to help, I can simply click a button, say the word, and hey presto the computer has done it for me.

◇ Typing is not for everyone. Some people just don't get on with it. Others may have conditions such as dyspraxia that prevent them becoming fluent enough at typing for it to be helpful. When I was at school speech recognition was expensive, time consuming to calibrate and inaccurate. Today it is part of everyday life. It is about as inclusive as assistive technology gets because using it is not special. People use their voice to write text messages when their hands are busy. You can even find out cinema times or order your shopping through your smart speaker.

◇ We take for granted the predictive text that is usually the default on our phones and in messenger apps. So long as you know the start of the word, it can be a great help to overcome difficulties with spelling. There are a range of free and affordable apps that can be downloaded that give you predictive text functionality.

◇ The literacy challenges of dyslexia are well known. The challenges with organising, managing time, focusing and getting things done are far less understood by many. These difficulties can have a much greater impact on school, work and personal life. The following points are all common features (known as productivity tools) of mainstream technology that can be incredibly enabling if a young person is shown how to use them and is supported to do so:

   - to-do lists

   - calendars and reminders

   - keeping your documents, media and other work organised

   - access to important information anytime, anywhere on any device.

◇ There are also several very powerful mobile apps which can enable your young person to use their phone camera to have text read to them.

I've learned a great deal about how to reduce the most difficult aspects of my own dyslexia and used this to help my own learners. I hope that these top tips are helpful to you and at least send you in the right direction to find more information to support your young person.

🔖 Key takeaways

- Everyone supporting a child with dyslexia should seek to really understand all their strengths and areas of challenge. This includes family, school staff, and most of all, the young person themselves.

- Build on the individual's strengths and interests. It can help shore up their self-esteem and resilience when they are finding other stuff difficult. It can help turn, 'I'm stupid and worthless' into, 'This thing is difficult right now'.

- Role models can help raise aspirations and show dyslexia is not going to be the thing that stops them succeeding. There are hundreds of famous examples, but it could just as easily be a teacher or family member.

- Dyslexia doesn't mean you can't love language.

- Find coping strategies that work for the individual.

CHAPTER 4

Identifying Signs of Dyslexia

BRITISH DYSLEXIA ASSOCIATION

Summary

◇ Indicators of dyslexia.

◇ Checklists and how they can help.

◇ Other factors that may result in indicators of dyslexia.

◇ The benefits and limitations of online screeners.

◇ Next steps.

Dyslexia is very common: 10–15 per cent of people will have dyslexia. However, many of those people will not know they have dyslexia, and most will not have a formal diagnosis. In the UK over 80 per cent of people with dyslexia leave school without a diagnosis. There are a variety of reasons for this.

First, dyslexia exists on a scale ranging from severe (around 4 per cent of the population) to moderate and mild. Those with mild dyslexia are often missed because simply the challenges their dyslexia presents are not particularly pronounced and the young person muddles through, naturally developing coping strategies that mask their dyslexia even further.

Second, it is all too often attributed to lower overall ability. Our school system, especially in primary school, measures young people's ability through their literacy (how they are progressing with reading and writing) and knowledge (learning times tables, names of places, dates, so on). It doesn't tend to look that closely at ability to solve problems, understand ideas or demonstrate verbal communications skills; these are areas in which young people with dyslexia are more likely to be able to display their natural aptitude. This means that someone who is struggling at school because of specific challenges related to dyslexia is often wrongly labelled as generally having low ability. The result of that can be tragic, the young person's potential is missed, and they are put on a life path that does not reflect what they have to offer the world.

The reality is that most teachers have received little or no formal training in spotting the signs of dyslexia. That is exacerbated by having to manage a large class. So you as a parent have a vital role in spotting the signs of dyslexia in your child.

In this chapter we will discuss what those signs are and how to explore in more detail whether your child is likely to have dyslexia. It should be noted that this is only the beginning of the journey; if the steps outlined in this chapter lead you to believe your child may be dyslexic, the next and crucial step is to get a Diagnostic Assessment (which is discussed in detail in the next chapter).

Dyslexia, although it is only part of an individual, is a big label to apply and will mean their life is different in many ways. Wrongly applying it must be avoided and, as we discuss in this chapter, indicators of dyslexia can have many causes, so do not assume that these mean dyslexia.

The other reason why this is only the start of the journey is that knowing your child is dyslexic is only part of the picture. If your child is to have the best opportunity to fulfil their potential, then you, they and their school must fully understand specifically how dyslexia affects them, their wider abilities and the specific support that they need.

Dyslexia checklists

The following are checklists of behaviours, abilities and circumstances that may be signs of dyslexia.[1] There is one for a child under six years old, one for primary and one for secondary aged children. Choose the one that is right for our child's age.

These checklists are from the BDA's *Dyslexia Friendly Schools Good Practice Guide* (Eastap and Gregory 2018). They are a useful tool to help parents spot areas of difficulty and strength which may indicate a child has dyslexia. For instance, if your child has a lot more 'yes's than 'no's in the difficulties sections, then you might consider speaking to a specialist, or seeking a formal assessment.

As you will see, the checklists don't just look at literacy issues and they include strengths. This is because, as we have discussed in previous chapters, dyslexia is not just about literacy challenges (although if your child is struggling with literacy development you should definitely explore whether dyslexia is a factor). What you will also note is that many of the things on the lists could be caused by many factors, so it is important not to leap to dyslexia based on one or two 'yes's.

You should also consider the severity of each of the areas;

---

1 These checklists are available to download from www.jkp.com/catalogue/book/9781787754263.

do not just assume that because your child really struggles with a few areas but not others, there is not something going on. The checklists are not a substitute for an assessment, but they can be a useful tool in thinking about things that can help your child and what areas they need more support in – interventions – and are something you could consider sharing with your child's school. You can also come to an organisation like the British Dyslexia Association, or a qualified assessor, although any assessment of your child will have a cost.

TWO TO SIX YEARS OLD

Difficulties	Yes	No
Family history of similar difficulties		
May have walked early but did not crawl		
History of intermittent hearing problems		
Difficulty in getting dressed, buttons, shoelaces		
Can be clumsy and show a lack of coordination		
Slow to develop speech		
Speech may be indistinct		
Problems finding the right word to describe things		
Difficulty in pronouncing long (multi-syllabic) words		
Lack of awareness of rhyme		
Lack of awareness of sounds in words		
Difficulty with naming letters		
Little interest in print/avoidance of reading		
Inability to read cvc words[2]		
Enjoys being read to, but can lose the thread of a story		

---

2   A consonant vowel consonant (cvc) word is a short word which is learnt at an early stage in reading such as cat, dog, sit, pet, dug.

Difficulty in following instructions		
Poor concentration		
Seems to tire quickly		
Has difficulty with social interactions with peers/adults		
Can be oversensitive		
Strengths		
Good receptive vocabulary		
Imaginative		
Enjoys practical activities – construction toys, etc.		
Enjoys conversation		
Empathetic to the needs/feelings of others		
Enjoys solving problems		
Interested in finding things out		
Good comprehension of texts when read to		
Prefers drawing pictures to writing		

Score:

PRIMARY AGE

Difficulties	Yes	No
Family history of similar difficulties		
Difficulty with phonological awareness, especially at the phoneme level		
Difficulty with following instructions		
Need for time to produce an oral response when questioned		
Lack of fluency in reading affecting comprehension		
Inaccurate decoding		
Fear of reading aloud		

cont.

Difficulties	Yes	No
A lack of enjoyment of reading		
Persistent and marked difficulty with spelling		
Messy, laboured handwriting		
Difficulty in finding the right word to describe things		
Mispronounces words		
Difficulty in remembering sequential information, e.g. alphabet, times tables, days of week		
Poor short-term working memory		
Takes longer than average to complete written tasks		
Difficulty copying from the board		
May describe visual discomfort when reading text		
Can be clumsy and lack coordination		
Mixing up numerical symbols		
Difficulty with maths vocabulary		
Miswriting of numbers		
Low self-esteem		
Behavioural difficulties		
Strengths		
Imaginative		
Good at thinking and reasoning skills		
Able to see the 'big picture'		
Good at problem solving		
Good general knowledge		
Good understanding of texts that have been read to him/her		
Curious		
Sophisticated receptive language		
Good visual-spatial skills		

Score:

SECONDARY AGE

Difficulties	Yes	No
Family history of similar difficulties		
Problems recalling facts		
Difficulty with recalling/following instructions		
Difficulty remembering sequential information, e.g. times tables, science procedures, historical facts		
Poor concept of time		
Problems with note taking		
Organisational difficulties, remembering homework, equipment, etc.		
Word finding difficulties		
Difficulty with fluent, accurate reading affecting comprehension		
Difficulty with/avoids reading aloud in class		
Difficulty with phonological awareness, especially at phonemic level		
Persistent difficulty with spelling		
Poor structure and organisation of written work		
Difficulty copying from the board		
Difficulty producing clear, legible handwriting		
Low self-esteem		
Aggressive or non-compliant behaviour		
Work avoidance tactics		
Lack of confidence		
Strengths		
Sophisticated receptive vocabulary		
Good critical thinking and reasoning skills		
Capacity to perceive information three-dimensionally		
Creative, imaginative, practical skills		

cont.

Strengths	Yes	No
Good interpersonal skills		
Intuitive		
Visual-spatial skills		
Good visual memory		
Capacity to see the 'big picture'		
Good general knowledge		
Sport and/or drama skills		

Score:

Other factors to consider

There are many things that can look like dyslexia but are not. You do not need to worry about this overly, as when you go for a Diagnostic Assessment, the assessor will look extensively at this to ensure they correctly diagnose dyslexia. However, it is worth being aware of some common reasons a young person can show signs of dyslexia but not in fact be dyslexic.

◇ **Physical factors**: It is always advisable to rule out any other physical factors such as previously undiagnosed problems with hearing or eyesight. In fact, an assessor will insist that your child has an up-to-date hearing and eye test before a Diagnostic Assessment.

◇ **Inadequate education**: If an individual has had limited opportunity to access education then it would not be surprising that their literacy levels may be lower than expected.

- ◇ **Broken or disrupted education**: If an individual has encountered frequent changes in education, such as frequent changes of school, it may also result in lower than expected literacy levels.

- ◇ **Disrupted social background**: If there is a history of social disruption, this may have had an impact on an individual in terms of them being receptive to education due to emotional upheaval.

- ◇ **People of lower ability levels**: Individuals who are of lower overall intellectual ability may well exhibit indicators that are similar to those of dyslexia, for example poor literacy or numeracy skills and difficulty with acquiring skills. Although this is not to say that someone of lower overall ability cannot also be dyslexic.

- ◇ **People who have suffered a brain injury**: In some circumstances damage to the brain sustained through an injury can also present in a very similar way to dyslexia.

- ◇ **Prescription medication**: Some prescription medication can affect the processing activities of the brain.

Online screeners

If, after completing a checklist and looking at other factors, you think your child may be dyslexic, then it may be a good next step to get some more information through an online screening test. However, you can, and it is perfectly usual to, go straight on to having a full Diagnostic Assessment.

Where an online screener may be particularly useful is

if you would like to take your concerns about your child's dyslexia to their school without incurring the cost of a full Diagnostic Assessment (£400 to £900). It may be that when presented with the result from a screener the school take steps themselves.

So, what is a screener? A good place to find an appropriate screener is the British Dyslexia Association website[3] which lists many that are of good standard and effective if administered correctly.

Whilst some screeners include checklist questions similar to those earlier in this chapter, they will also put your child through a range of tests (this will vary depending on the screener and age range it is designed for) and, based on your child's scores, they will flag results that may indicate dyslexia. Most, especially those for younger children, are designed to be enjoyable for the child and will typically take much less than hour to complete. They also tend to cost very little.

If you are administering a screener at home, be careful to read the instructions carefully. How you administer the test can have a massive impact on the results, so whilst detailed instructions can be a frustration to plough through, it is worth doing so on this occasion.

You will often see tutors and charities running cheap or even free screening for dyslexia. This can often be very good but be cautious. Remember that whilst a Diagnostic Assessment is heavily regulated and must be carried out by a highly qualified professional, no such regulation exists with screening. If in doubt, take a look at the British Dyslexia Association website for more details.

---

3   www.bdadyslexia.org.uk.

Whilst they are certainly not a replacement for a Diagnostic Assessment, screeners are an immediate and cheap way of getting a better picture of your child and can add helpful context in conversations with schools.

Next steps

Based on a checklist or screener or both, if you think your child may have dyslexia, what is the next step?

That is very simple: you need to get a full Diagnostic Assessment, which we discuss in detail in the next chapter.

A word of warning here: this is likely to have a cost – at least £400. Whilst the British Dyslexia Association campaigns hard for Diagnostic Assessments to be freely available through schools, it is unlikely (although not impossible) that your school will cover this cost. We appreciate for any family this is a large amount of money and for many, a barrier.

Financial burden aside, it is important to remember a diagnosis of dyslexia is a positive step. Dyslexia is a difference in how the brain processes information and in the right environment it can be immensely powerful. Your child is taking the first step on a path that, although often frustrating and difficult, has the potential to take them on to amazing opportunities, and lead a successful and fulfilling life.

Key takeaways

- There are many indicators of dyslexia, which can sometimes be missed or misinterpreted.

- Indicators of dyslexia don't mean your child is dyslexic; you need a full Diagnostic Assessment to confirm dyslexia.

- Checklists are a good place to start to find out if your child may be dyslexic.

- There are other factors that could cause signs of dyslexia, so be careful to consider these.

- Online screening tools can be helpful to give you a better picture, but they are not infallible.

Reference

Eastap, L. & Gregory, J. (2018) *Dyslexia Friendly Schools Good Practice Guide*. London: British Dyslexia Association.

CHAPTER 5

How Dyslexia Is Diagnosed and Why It Is Important

KATRINA COCHRANE

Summary

◇ What is a Diagnostic Assessment and what does it entail?

◇ Who can carry out a Diagnostic Assessment?

◇ What happens before a Diagnostic Assessment?

◇ The outcomes, information and recommendations from a Diagnostic Assessment.

◇ Next steps after a Diagnostic Assessment.

If you think your child may have dyslexia, then you will have come across terms like 'dyslexia assessment' or 'getting a diagnosis'. These refer to what is known as a Diagnostic Assessment.

A Diagnostic Assessment means something very specific. The tests carried out, the qualifications of the assessors and the areas covered in the report are all stipulated and regulated by an accrediting body (called the Standards of Assessment in SpLD Committee or SASC for short). It is the only way to get a definitive diagnosis for dyslexia.

Most importantly, it is the first step in understanding your child's dyslexia. A Diagnostic Assessment doesn't just rule out other reasons your child may have challenges that indicate dyslexia; the range of tests and the experience of an expert mean you can get a full picture of the specific ways it manifests, their underlying cognitive abilities, any co-occurring conditions, and specific support strategies that might help them.

Whilst it is an intense experience for a young person, half a day of testing and questions, and it is often a substantial financial investment, it very important that any young person who shows indicators of dyslexia receives a Diagnostic Assessment. A full Diagnostic Assessment should not be confused with screeners and checklists, which we discuss in Chapter 4.

What is the difference between an assessment with an Educational Psychologist and an assessment with a Specialist Dyslexia Assessor?

The first decision you have to make about a Diagnostic Assessment is whether it is carried out by an Educational Psychologist (EP) or a Specialist Dyslexia Assessor. Both are able to diagnose dyslexia; the assessment they carry out is the same and their report has the same legal standing. In practice, either will do an excellent job and there is little to choose between them. However, there are a few factors to consider.

◇ As a rule of thumb, an EP is the best option for assessments where the child has complex needs; a Specialist Dyslexia Assessor, who may have spent longer in the classroom, would be better for practical strategies that you and your child's school can put into action.

◇ Educational Psychologists have access to a different type of test which Specialist Dyslexia Assessors are not able to use. Although they may be a specialist in dyslexia, they are likely to have experience across a range of learning differences and developmental challenges.

◇ A Specialist Dyslexia Assessor will likely have more experience of classroom teaching and directly supporting dyslexic learners. This means they may have more practical experience of delivering the support strategies they are recommending, which can make the report more practical and helpful for both parent and classroom teacher.

◇ Another factor to consider is cost. An EP is likely to charge at the upper end of the cost band mentioned in Chapter 4, so in the region of £750 to £1000 for a Diagnostic Assessment but a Specialist Dyslexia Assessor will charge between around £400 and £600.

What is the difference between a Diagnostic Assessment and tests for Exam Access Arrangements?

Tests carried out for Exam Access Arrangements are designed to identify if individuals need any additional support in exams, such as more time or the use of a scribe. The tests used are the same as some of the tests used in a Diagnostic Assessment, but those used for Exam Access Arrangements will not come up with a diagnosis of any Specific Learning Difficulty.

They are not interested in the reason for the need, which could be dyslexia but could be a wide range of things; they are just checking if the child has a need for access arrangements which will help them achieve their potential in, for example, their GCSEs.

What to check before the assessment takes place

Diagnostic Assessments should always be conducted by a certified person, qualified to assess. This could be:

- ◇ a Chartered Psychologist specialising in Specific Learning Difficulties registered with the Health Care Practitioners Council (HCPC)

- ◇ a Specialist Teacher/Assessor with an Assessment Practising Certificate (APC) issued by one of the three providers, i.e. British Dyslexia Association, Dyslexia Action or PATOSS. These need to be renewed every three years.

Data privacy

Before the assessment the parent or carer will sign a privacy notice that means that they understand where the report will be stored, for how long, and who will have access to it. This may be a tick to consent on a website or a paper copy signed to comply with GDPR.

Both EPs and Specialist Dyslexia Assessors should have indemnity insurance and DBS checks in place if they are working with children.

Covid-19

At the time of writing, many safety precautions have been put in place due to Covid-19; you may be asked to bring along your own pens and paper, for example. Social distancing will of course be observed, and you should also be given a short risk assessment to sign before the assessment.

How to book a Diagnostic Assessment

The British Dyslexia Association website has information about Diagnostic Assessments and how to get an assessment.[1]

Before the Diagnostic Assessment takes place

The assessor will spend time collating information about your child before the Diagnostic Assessment. This will be gathered from a variety of sources so that a fully holistic understanding of your child is captured. The assessor will want to gather this information from the individual themselves, teachers and SENCOs, as well as parents or carers. They will be sensitive about what information is recorded and make sure that it is used only for the purposes of the assessment itself.

---

1 www.bdadyslexia.org.uk/services/assessments/diagnostic-assessments.

Information from your child's school

The assessor will ask wide range of questions to your child's teachers and SENCO to get a picture of their performance in school via a pre-assessment questionnaire.

If the assessor is carrying out the assessment in school they will talk directly to teachers and teaching assistants and to the SENCO, as well as collecting some of the information by way of questionnaires. Information collected from your child's school will include whether your child passed the phonics test and what their National Curriculum Attainment Levels are.

Some assessors may observe a lesson or look at the child's school work, but this is not always the case.

Information the assessor will need from you

The assessor will need some background information from you about your child. Questions may be asked about the birth, such as whether it was a full-term pregnancy, for example. Other questions may relate to your child's developmental history and, typically, questions about developmental milestones associated with language and physical development will be asked. They will also check for any history of hearing or visual difficulties, as well as information about fine motor skills such as handwriting.

A recent hearing and eye test will be required before the assessment and a visual difficulties questionnaire will be circulated, as the assessor may advise an optometrist appointment. If your child wears glasses or uses a specific colour overlay as their normal way of working they should bring them to the assessment. If they are on any relevant medication this should be noted in advance and it should be taken as normal.

The assessor will ask for information about your child's language development and the ease or difficulty with which they acquired literacy skills. There may have been previous speech and language (or occupational) therapy and information on this will need to be passed on.

They will ask about your child's experience of school and the kind of teaching that they have been exposed to. Have they had any additional learning support in the past and, if so, what did this entail and how useful was it?

They will also want to know if English is the only language spoken at home. If it is not, then the assessor may not wish to assess the child, unless the child has lived in the UK for a significant period of time. The assessor will ask if there are any literacy challenges in the rest of the family and these will be noted, but confidentially.

The assessor will want to capture a picture of your child's family and home life (without being intrusive) and how, if any, circumstances might have affected their learning – for instance, missing school during the Covid-19 pandemic lockdowns in 2020 and 2021.

They will want to gather an idea of whether or not school is enjoyable or stressful, information about their memory, communication skills and social interaction, as well as what they have interests in, and how they might spend their leisure time. What are their plans for the future and what do they perceive to be their strengths?

In the questionnaire, questions may also be asked about friendship groups and how they are perceived by their peers.

What a Diagnostic Assessment involves

A Diagnostic Assessment will involve a series of tests that will give a profile of the individual's strengths and limitations in a number of key areas of cognitive ability:

◇ verbal and non-verbal (visual) ability

◇ short-term and working memory – the ability to retain and use information held in memory

◇ phonological awareness – the ability to understand and apply knowledge of sounds, i.e. to generate rhyming words or 'sound out' unknown words when reading

◇ speed of processing – being able to quickly and accurately 'pull' information from long-term memory, such as the meanings of words.

The assessment will also involve age-appropriate tests that measure attainment in reading, spelling and writing.

Normally, an assessment will take around two-and-a-half hours, but the assessor will go at your child's speed and allow plenty of breaks. For post-16-year-olds it is likely to take around three hours to take into account additional tests needed for adults. Generally, most children enjoy the whole process and are quite happy to be tested.

The assessor is trying to find out what discrepancy there is between the child's potential to learn (underlying ability) and the rest of the tests carried out. Most dyslexic children have average or above-average verbal or visual abilities but show a difference between these and the rest of the tests. It is worth noting that according to the Rose

Report (2009), dyslexia can occur at any level of intellectual ability.

Underlying ability

The child will be given a battery of both verbal and non-verbal/visual tasks and many children with dyslexia show a discrepancy between and within these sub-tests. They will be asked questions to check their level of vocabulary and also timed construction tasks to show visual skills. Children with dyspraxia often find these latter tasks difficult as they have weak abilities in spatial awareness.

Memory and processing

A child with dyslexia will often have challenges with short-term and working memory. Their speed of processing verbal or visual information may also be impaired.

In a test of repeating increasing digits and letters, the assessor will assess short-term auditory memory. Holding those numbers and letters in their head and manipulating them to repeat them backwards will assess working memory. These skills are important in the classroom where children will have difficulty remembering oral instructions or remembering things like their times tables.

The ability to process information efficiently is often measured by the rapid verbal naming of items presented visually, such as a series of random letters or numbers. Children who find such tasks difficult may find it hard to work at the same speed as their peers.

Reading

This will assess a variety of skills required for full fluency. At the very least, single word reading, non-word reading and reading comprehension will be explored. The assessment might also involve a listening comprehension, an oral reading comprehension or a silent reading comprehension. Reading speed or rate may also be recorded. For the younger child their knowledge of sound–symbol correspondence may be tested.

Observations will be made, for example, if your child uses their finger to help them track the text, and if they miss out words or letters.

Spelling

This will be in the form of an age-appropriate single word test, but throughout the assessment there will be other chances for the assessor to look at spellings, such as in the free writing task, or in any school work that has been provided.

Writing

Free writing (for example, writing about their family or their pets) provides an opportunity for the child being assessed to show their ability to express themselves in written form. For post-16 assessment a more academic extended piece of writing is required.

The assessor will observe their pen grip, which hand they use, their ability to put down their ideas on paper, the quality of content in the writing, the level of vocabulary used, as well as fluency of expression. Many individuals with dyslexic traits have vivid and innovative ideas but find it difficult to express these in written form. Is there a discrepancy, for instance, between their written and spoken skills?

This exercise also provides a chance to examine how the individual executes the writing. Do they, for example, produce letters that are neatly formed, or is the writing messy and difficult to read? Do they use a pen with relative ease and dexterity, or do they hold their pen in an unusual or awkward way?

The free writing will be completed within a time limit, so that speed of handwriting is also assessed, although it is also usual for a separate speed of copying test to accompany the free writing exercise.

Other areas

In addition to the core tests, the assessor might also explore other areas, such as motor coordination, or record any evidence of visual difficulties. They may also test mathematical skills.

After the Diagnostic Assessment

You may be offered some verbal feedback immediately after the assessment, but sometimes the assessor needs to go away and think about all the test scores before coming to a conclusion. You should be offered the opportunity to discuss the written report when you receive it, which should be within two to three weeks of the assessment. The report will be sent to you with password protected access in order to comply with Data Protection Regulations.

You should make an appointment and take the report into the SENCO at your child's school. It may be best to take out the most important points and summarise them or turn them into bullet points of strengths and limitations so that these can be shared with the relevant staff quickly.

Diagnostic Assessment report

The outcome and results will be different for every person and the assessment will produce a unique profile, in the form of a written report. The report should be clearly written with accessible language that makes transparent the areas in which the individual has strengths, as well as limitations, in a holistic and accessible format. It should also contain very clear guidelines and suggestions for structured and well-tested interventions so that teachers, parents and the individual themselves have a very clear understanding of the way forward.

The recommendations should be clearly set out under targeted headings, like the ones suggested below:

◇ specialist teaching and support

◇ classroom/mainstream/general academic support and adjustments

◇ assistive technology or resources that might help

◇ Exam Access Arrangements (final decision on these is up to the school)

◇ strategies that might help at home

◇ future considerations – especially when transition is to

be made to secondary school or further or higher education

◇ any further referrals.

Further referrals

There may be a referral to a paediatric occupational therapist (OT) if, for example, dyspraxia is suspected. In addition, there may be referrals made to behavioural optometrists if visual difficulties are present. The person being assessed may also be referred to the GP for possible attention deficit disorder or autistic difficulties as these can co-occur with dyslexia.

Interpreting the report

Your report may show the test results using a graph and you will be able to see the 'spiky profile' normally associated with a specific learning difficulty. Here there will be peaks and troughs where your child has strengths as well as limitations.

The results will be reported in Standard Scores, which are calculated by taking the raw score and transforming it into a common scale. A Standard Score between 90 and 110 is within the mid-average range. You may see a discrepancy between some scores, and for the dyslexic child this is normal as they have strengths in some areas such as vocabulary but relative weaknesses in other areas assessed, including attainment. You may also see percentile scores discussed. These compare your child's score with a hundred children of the same age where the 50th percentile is the mid-point score and is within the average range. This is equivalent to a Standard Score of 100, which is the mid-point of the Standard Score range.

How the report is structured

The report you receive will have a detachable summary at the beginning of the report which will give a diagnostic decision about your child. At the back of the report will be a list of recommendations and a summary table of results. You will be encouraged to show the report to your child's school and these recommendations will hopefully be taken on board.

What kind of recommendations might be made?

These vary according to the age and individual needs of the child but will generally include some recommendations for a teaching programme that is structured, cumulative and multisensory.

For the child who has difficulty writing quickly and legibly, touch typing is often recommended using a programme like Touch-type Read & Spell (TTRS) so that using a laptop becomes their 'normal way of working'.

Other recommendations might be for Exam Access Arrangements, such as additional time or a reader or scribe. These ultimately will be up to the school to decide according to the child's normal way of working.

Explaining the diagnosis to your child

It is very important that your child is made aware of the whole process and what it actually means. The assessor will ask your child how they feel about their difficulties and the child's voice is an important part of the assessment report. The results of the testing should be shared with your child as it may help improve their motivation and self-esteem.

Working with your child's school after the Diagnostic Assessment

Recommendations for class teachers may include:

◇ giving fewer verbal instructions and breaking information down into smaller steps

◇ less copying from the whiteboard

◇ help with putting homework in planners

◇ working with a TA or specialist teacher on a structured, cumulative and multisensory teaching programme

◇ using assistive technology.

For older children there may be suggestions for study skills to help with organisation and planning, reading techniques and exam strategies.

A school may not take on board the recommendations of a privately commissioned report, but most do. You can find out more about what to do if your child's school is refusing to accept a Diagnostic Assessment Report on the British Dyslexia Association website.[2]

---

2 www.bdadyslexia.org.uk.

Disabled Students Allowance

In time your child may go to university and the report will be able to be used to apply for Disabled Students Allowance (DSA) through Student Finance[3] if the assessor had a current APC (or was HCPC registered) at time of writing the report.[4]

Key takeaways

- Diagnostic Assessments are the only way to get a definitive diagnosis of dyslexia.

- Assessors gather a wide range of information ahead of and make observations during the Diagnostic Assessment to get a full picture of the child.

- A range of tests are carried out during Diagnostic Assessments to understand the depth and breadth of your child's strengths and weaknesses.

- From the Diagnostic Assessment you will get a detailed report with recommendations about next steps and support strategies.

Reference

Rose, J. (2009) *Identifying and Teaching Children and Young People with Dyslexia and Literacy Difficulties.* Nottingham: DCSF.

---

3   https://www.gov.uk/student-finance (England); https://www.student financewales.co.uk (Wales); https://www.mygov.scot/apply-student-loan (Scotland); https://www.studentfinanceni.co.uk (Northern Ireland).
4   You can check if an APC is current by going to www.sasc.org.uk.

CHAPTER 6

Supporting Children's Literacy Development

BRITISH DYSLEXIA ASSOCIATION

Summary

◇ What the elements of literacy learning are.

◇ Why phonological awareness is important and how you can support your child to develop it.

◇ Progressing to reading.

◇ Developing writing skills for young people with dyslexia.

◇ A word or two about spelling.

In this chapter, we will look at one of the key areas young people with dyslexia are likely to struggle with – developing literacy.

It takes many months and years of study to become an expert in supporting literacy for young people with dyslexia and it is totally natural to feel overwhelmed about how best to support your child in this area. That is why we have educational professionals.

This may be exacerbated by your own dyslexia. Many of

the areas we discuss in this chapter are a real struggle for adults with dyslexia, regardless of how bright they are or what support they may have received with their dyslexia. So, do not feel bad if you have a practical or psychological barrier with supporting your dyslexic child's literacy development; you are not unusual.

However, it is useful to understand the principles of how literacy learning develops over time and know about some practical activities that you may want to use to support your child develop their skills. So that is what we will discuss in this chapter.

Do not stress if your child really struggles with some or many of the things in this chapter. Dyslexia can make literacy much harder, but is crucial to always remember that it does not affect your child's underlying ability and can bring many strengths, which we discuss in more detail elsewhere. Dyslexia is not a barrier to success.

Also, ensure that you get the professional support that is out there. Primary teachers, even if they are not experts in dyslexia, will be experts in teaching phonics. There are also many excellent resources and technology programmes available produced by experts. The British Dyslexia Association website[1] is a good place to start to look for these. And, if you can afford it, there are excellent dyslexia specialists out there who can provide direct support for your child.

Phonological awareness

The awareness of sounds in language is an important starting point to enable success in learning to read and spell.

---

1   www.bdadyslexia.org.uk.

This awareness of the sounds in language is known as 'phonological awareness'. Phonological awareness is covered in several chapters in the book, but explored in more depth in this chapter.

Research tells us that this can be a particularly challenging area for dyslexic children because of the direct impact of their dyslexia on this area of skills development.

For reading, the written letters represent the sound to be produced (decoding) and for spelling the sounds in the word are matched to the letters and then written down (encoding). In both encoding and decoding, phonological awareness is needed because the individual must recognise the sounds (and be able to segment them) in the words in order to link them to the letters.

We will look at the core elements of phonological awareness and ideas for activities to build these with your child. The elements we are going to look at are:

◇ sequencing

◇ syllables

◇ rhyme

◇ segmenting sounds

◇ vocabulary development

◇ phonics

◇ blending sounds together

◇ dealing with longer words.

It is worth noting here that it is important, where possible, to have an individual's hearing assessed. Clearly if an individual cannot hear the sounds in words because of a hearing difficulty then it is likely that they may have problems discriminating sounds, particularly where the sounds are very similar.

Sequencing activities

One of the first parts in the process of developing phonological skills is to be able to sequence words and/or sounds in a set order. Sequencing can be a challenge for dyslexic individuals so is worth practising.

Activities to support this area could include:

◇ While reading a story give the child a sequence of pictures that they can hold up as the story is read. After listening to the story ask them to then replicate the sequence of the story and recount the key events that relate to each picture.

◇ Children can be given pictures in a random order that would form a story. They then sequence the pictures to make the story and recount the story verbally.

◇ Simple games such as 'Simon says...' or 'I went to the shops and bought...' are also helpful with a group of children. For example, the first child starts by saying 'I went to the shops and bought some bread', followed by the next child who adds to the list with 'I went to the shops and bought some bread and some milk' and so on, going around the group until the list becomes too long to remember. Then the game can start again.

Any activity that encourages the child to reproduce a sequence is helpful for this area of skills development.

Syllable counting

Phonological awareness develops along a scale of increasing difficulty, with larger sound units, such as the word and syllable, developed before smaller units, such as the individual letter sound.

Activities to support this area of development might include:

- ◇ Collect a bag of small items or toys and place them in a feely bag (a feely bag is a small cloth bag; it is important that the child cannot see the contents of the bag). Make sure you have items in your bag that cover one, two and three syllable words and perhaps even four syllable words. Tell the child that words have beats in them, like music. Listen to the beats in this word 'ba-na-na'. Tap your hand on the floor and beat out the syllables in the word, saying the word slowly. Alternatively place your hand under your chin; each time your chin touches your hand this is a syllable or a beat in a word. Pass the bag to the child and have them select an item or toy. The child says what the item is, then taps out the drumbeats on the floor.

- ◇ **Syllable hoops**: Lay out three or four hoops on the floor. These will be used for the child to jump into when they break up a word into its syllables. Read a word out loud. The child then repeats the word and as they say each syllable, they jump into a hoop.

- ◇ This can also be done verbally by using some words that are of interest to the child, for example, how many syllables in Everton, Chelsea, Leeds, etc. Such activities can be extended by asking the child to think of their own words with a set number of syllables in them.

Activities that involve a number are also easy to convert to board games. For example, the child could turn over a picture playing card and count/beat the number of syllables to allow their move on the board game (e.g. tel-e-vi-sion would be four moves).

Rhyme

Rhyme is often something that individuals with phonological processing challenges may struggle with, including:

- ◇ **Recognition**: 'Does hat rhyme with cat?', 'Does fun rhyme with dog?'

- ◇ **Matching**: Choice of three pictures, child is asked to find the two that rhyme.

- ◇ **Odd one out**: Three pictures, child has to find the one that doesn't rhyme.

- ◇ **Roll a rhyme**: Make up some dice that have rhyming words on them and the pairs of dice are matched according to the rhyming words that appear on them. Roll the dice together, say the words and decide if they rhyme.

- ◇ **Games with rhyming cards**: Use picture cards that include multiple examples of rhyming words, for example, 'at', 'an' word families. Use about four word families. The aim is to build up a pile of cards that match with each rhyming pattern.

Once the child can match rhyming words and identify the odd one out, they are ready to move into the production of rhyme.

Activities could include:

◇ **Silly poems**: Make up nonsense poems using the same rhyming sound, for example:

  - The rat wearing a h...(hat)

  - Went and sat on the m...(mat).

◇ **The ship is loaded with...** (from *Phonemic Awareness in Young Children*, Adams 1998): Seat the children in a circle and have a bean bag or ball to toss. To begin the game, say, 'The ship is loaded with cheese.' Then toss the ball to somebody in the circle. This person must produce a rhyme, for example, 'The ship is loaded with *peas*' and throw the ball back to you. Repeating your original rhyme, then toss the ball to another child. Continue the game in this way until they run out of rhymes. Then begin the game with new cargo, for example, 'The ship is loaded with (dogs, hogs, frogs, etc).'

◇ For older children, looking at poems, song lyrics or raps can also be useful for developing these skills in an interesting way. Alternatively, a selection of rhyming words can be given, and the child asked to develop their own lyric, rap or poem; internet sites such as rhymezone.com can be very helpful to generate ideas. Work by Katie Overy *et al.* (2003) and Usha Goswami (2019) has identified that musical activities can also be helpful in developing these skills.

Segmenting sounds

This is the ability to identify individual sounds in words and separate them out. Skills can be developed in a structured way, starting with the easiest then moving to the more challenging sounds.

- ◇ **Recognition**: 'Does cat start with the same sound as cup?'

- ◇ **Matching**: Choice of three pictures, child chooses the two that start with the same sound.

- ◇ **Odd one out**: 'Find the one that doesn't start with c.'

- ◇ **Production**: 'Tell me two words that start with c.'

Children need to be able to isolate sounds in words. Sounds are said quickly in speech, so it is important to use a multisensory approach when isolating sounds. This involves helping the child to understand how a sound feels when it is produced, along with understanding how the tongue and lips move when producing sounds.

Using a mirror can be helpful here so that the child can see what their mouth is doing when they make the sounds. It can also be helpful for them to describe what their mouth is doing by asking such questions as, 'What shape are your lips?'

Activities to help with sound recognition could include:

- ◇ **My pile your pile**: In this game the child is listening for a specific sound at the beginning of a word. Have a pile of approximately 12 picture cards. Six cards have pictures of things that start with the same sound; six cards have pictures that start with a different sound. Turn the cards over and ask the child what sound the word starts with (as represented by the picture). If they get it right, the card belongs to their pile, and if wrong, the card belongs to your pile.

⬦ **I spy**: 'Tell me something that starts with (letter sound)...'

⬦ **Books**: Select pictures from books you read to the child and have them:

- find something that starts with a particular sound

- point to a picture and tell you what sound the object (word) starts with.

Once the child can identify the initial sounds of words, they then need to move on to segmenting all the other sounds within short (and simple words). Segmenting words into individual sounds has a strong relationship to the development of spelling skills.

Many children will manage three sound words to start with (e.g. h-e-n), but you could start with two sounds such as up, it, etc.

Activities to help with segmentation could include:

⬦ Using a feely bag with items in it that have three sounds. The child brings out an item and has to say the sounds of the item they are holding.

⬦ The child could be asked to count the sounds in a word, without looking, and then compare it with the number of letters, to discover that it is not always the same.

⬦ A simple but effective activity is to ask the child to identify where in a word they hear a particular sound, for example, where do they hear the 'a' sound in ant (beginning), where in bat (middle) and where in the more complicated banana.

Understanding reading

Reading is a skill to be learned; children do not naturally translate marks on paper into words and meaning.

Reading requires a combination of skills. Most of these are automatic to good readers, enabling them to concentrate on the meaning and only have to think about the mechanics of reading when they come across a word that is unknown.

For some dyslexic individuals cracking the reading code can take a great deal more effort and practice and in turn, therefore, take a lot longer to achieve the level of competence that enables an individual to extract meaning from what they have read.

Often for the dyslexic child, the act of reading is so difficult that they really struggle to get any meaning from what they have read easily. Therefore, there is no 'reward'. Dyslexic children often do not read for pleasure; it is simply too difficult and too much hard work.

Vocabulary development

If a child is not reading at an age-appropriate level, this can also impact negatively on vocabulary development. It is therefore important for vocabulary development to be seen as a different and separate skill to reading that needs to be developed.

Making use of audiobooks and having detailed discussions are really important for dyslexic children so that they are able to develop a good level of vocabulary, even if they are not reading a lot or not reading at an age-appropriate level. Poor vocabulary will have a significant impact on the child's ability to express their thoughts and ideas and also on writing, so it is important that a lot of effort is dedicated to this area. Parents can play a key role in this.

Sharing audiobooks and then discussing them, looking at interesting images and describing them, watching films and talking about them, visiting places of interest and exploring ideas, thoughts and concepts are of vital importance, and a sound investment in the child's future.

It is also worth noting here that for some dyslexic children, particularly those with poor short-term memory, stories (fiction) may pose a range of additional challenges. This can be because they forget what is going on in a story, – by the time a page is completed they have forgotten who the characters are and what is going on, so the whole thing becomes rather pointless and they therefore might struggle to engage with stories very well.

In such cases nonfiction may be a far better option, particularly where the subject is of interest to the child. The connection of nonfiction to the real world is often far more engaging. It also provides the additional bonus that they are learning about other things.

It may also be worth considering encouraging the use of text reading software. This is now built into many word processing packages and can really help with accessing text efficiently, reading, researching and also proofreading.

Reading books that are sent home from school along with the 'reading record' to be completed can create significant problems for parents when the child does not want to read. This is an area where you really do need to discuss the issues with your child's teacher to find an alternative strategy where reading practice can happen, but in a way that works for everyone. This may be through games, nonfiction, or other activities instead.

Letter–sound correspondence (phonics)

English is basically an alphabetic–phonetic language. That is, the majority of words are made up of letters and letter-groups that represent sounds. Most words can be 'sounded out' with only a few completely irregular words that have to be learned. However, a reader has to learn quite a lot of letter combinations and their sounds in order to be efficient at phonic decoding.

Most children learn the letter–sound links for the basic five vowels and 21 consonants, and 'crack the code' in that way. The longer letter groups (sh, ee, ou, igh, etc.) are just 'picked up' by many children as they notice them in words. However, for struggling readers, these letter combinations may well need to be specifically taught.

The dyslexic child, even from the earliest stages of learning to read, can feel overwhelmed by the sheer volume of new information that is being delivered and the speed at which they are expected to move on. Failure to grasp these initial stages means that the child gets progressively left further behind and when new and more complex pieces of information are introduced the foundations are just not there and they soon begin to flounder.

READING CARDS
This is a simple technique that acts as an aide-memoire and a tool that can be used to practise letters and sounds with

the child. For each new reading skill that is taught, a small card (about the size of a business card) can be made and used as an aide-memoire. On the front of the card in the middle, the lower-case letter or group of letters can be written; in the bottom right-hand corner the upper case can be written. On the back of the card at the top a clue word can be written and next to it the sound in brackets (this shows that it is the sound), for example, gate (g).

The individual can be encouraged to draw a picture of the clue word as a reminder. Gradually a pack of reading cards can be built up as more sounds are added. These cards can also be used for high frequency words that can be put onto a different colour card. Vowels can also be put on a different colour card to help the child distinguish them easily.

The routine is that the child looks at the front of the card with the letter on, says the clue word first and then the sound, for example, gate (g). The cards need to be shuffled as the pack grows to ensure that they come in a random way. If the child cannot remember the sound, then they can check the picture on the reverse of the card to remind themselves. These cards should be practised as often as possible (ideally every day).

Depending on the child, an element of competition can be added, such as timing to see how fast they can go through the pack. Once you are certain that a sound is embedded that card can be removed from the pack; this can take a long time as the aim of this activity is to build links between the sound and the symbol without the child having to think about them.

For older children it is possible to do a computerised version of reading cards or put them onto a smartphone, which can save them feeling self-conscious.

Blending sounds into words

Once some basic letter and sound links are known, these letters need to be blended into words. Blending individual letters together to form words can pose great difficulty for some children. They might sound out the letters correctly but look blank when it comes to saying the actual word or indeed instead say something completely different. This can be the case particularly for those individuals with poor short-term memory.

Activities to help with blending might include:

◇ Using wooden or plastic letters and encouraging the child to physically move them together as they say them out loud.

◇ Tracing over each letter with a finger or pencil whilst sounding out, which also encourages them to remember the sounds by adding a kinaesthetic link.

◇ Cursive (joined up) handwriting. This can also be particularly helpful. The child should be encouraged to write the word whilst making the corresponding sounds. The physical links between each letter using cursive writing style encourages the child to prolong each sound in their mouth.

ROOT WORD SUFFIX OR PREFIX SEGMENTS
As skills improve, the child may encounter longer words, and then they need to have a strategy to break these longer words into more manageable chunks. Recognising suffixes and prefixes can be helpful.

As a definition a suffix is something that is added to a root word that changes its meaning. For example, adding the suffix 's' to a word usually makes it plural – there are more than one of that thing, for example, cat > cats. A prefix is added to the beginning of a word and also changes its meaning.

The good news about prefixes and suffixes is that they are often very straightforward, once you know how to recognise them, and many long words are simply a short root word with prefixes and suffixes added. There are many suffixes and prefixes and you can find lists of them on the internet. For older children it is also interesting to explore the meaning of suffixes and prefixes as this starts to develop a better understanding of how language works and develops vocabulary. For example, help – helpful – unhelpful – unhelpfully.

A useful activity here is to go through a piece of real text and identify the suffixes by putting a box around them; the same can be done with prefixes, which can be underlined or circled in a different colour. Using different colours can help this process and make these aspects of a word stand out more.

It is important to control the volume of suffixes being introduced. It is better to start with one or two at a time.

Activities to support this area of development could include:

◇ Simple activities such as playing longest word games. The child is given a simple base or root word and the task is to add as many prefixes and suffixes as possible, whilst still being able to read the word. It can also be useful to discuss the meaning of each suffix and prefix to explore how they change the meaning of the word and build vocabulary.

SYLLABLES

Longer words can also be split into syllables to make them accessible to read. The practice provided by syllable counting and identification activities discussed previously will help a child to identify syllables in words. Splitting up words into syllables often depends on where the vowel is in the syllables. There are several online videos that explain 'long and short vowels sound', 'open and closed syllables' and 'syllable division'. It is a good idea to have a look at some of these and watch demonstrations about how to tackle longer words using syllable division techniques.

Activities to support this area of development could include:

◇ Board games, which can be adapted to be used for literacy practice by adding in cards with words of varying syllable number on. The players place their counters on the board and move their counters the number of spaces that match the number of syllables in a word.

Writing

In simple terms the purpose of writing is to communicate with others to pass on information or to tell someone about something.

Writing is often something that a dyslexic child is reluctant to do. There are number of reasons for this.

◇ Writing is just generally hard. It is the bringing together of a whole range of skills, such as knowing and remembering what you want to write, finding the right words and sentences and holding them in short-term memory whilst you write them.

Then, while doing that, you have to know how to spell the words and know how to form the letters to write the words. There are multiple layers of skill that have to all come together in perfect harmony to produce a piece of written work. An additional challenge is if that piece of writing then has to conform to a particular format or style that may also be unfamiliar due to lack of reading experience.

◊ The other factor that causes anxiety is that once you have written something it is lasting evidence of how good or bad you are at writing. Then, often, other people judge you on this performance. For dyslexic children they are often well aware that what they produce in written form actually has little resemblance to what they know or how able they are, or indeed how much effort they have put into the task only then to come up short.

It is no wonder that dyslexic children are often reluctant to commit words to paper despite often having amazing ideas, high amounts of knowledge and a creative imagination.

Supporting dyslexic children with writing is therefore a challenge. This challenge is then increased further if the individual has not much experience of different types of writing because they lack good reading skills and therefore exposure to various different types of writing genres.

The way that we write in the modern world has changed dramatically – instead of formal letters we write informal emails, instead of writing letters to friends and family we use social media, instead of chatting we might text. The conventions are often very different between writing in day-to-day life and writing in education. It is not unusual for a child or young person to be an avid user of social media but a highly reluctant writer in school.

Any writing is good

For many reluctant writers any writing in any form that they do is good. A text message or social media post may not seem to have the same academic value as an essay, but for a dyslexic individual they have 'put themselves out there' and this has often taken a great deal of bravery. Of course, with social media there is the bonus of predictive text, which makes things a lot easier, but they will have still produced a written communication.

Using technology can be hugely helpful for a dyslexic child, as the functions of predictive text, spell checkers, and the ability to delete all make life easier. Typing removes the additional burden of having to recall the letter shapes and then form those shapes. The use of voice recognition software can also be a complete game changer for some individuals.

Handwriting versus typing

This is a complex debate and one that there simply is not enough time to explore in this chapter. Cursive (joined up) handwriting can be helpful for a dyslexic child to support things like spelling and blending sounds in words for reading. Using a fully joined up style can help to create a kinaesthetic memory for the word and help the sounds to be merged together as they write and say the words out loud, particularly high frequency words like 'said', 'the' and so on.

That said, if the 'act' of writing is creating an additional barrier where the individual is having to think so hard about the shape of a letter that they forget what they are writing, then using a keyboard may well be better and more efficient. If the decision is made to use a keyboard, then it is important that the individual learns to touch type in order that they can write efficiently. There are numerous touch typing programmes available and some of these are listed on the British Dyslexia Association website.[2] Most children can start to learn to touch type effectively from around the age of seven to eight years.

In simple terms, if the act of writing is getting in the way, then consider moving to working on a keyboard instead. This is not an easy decision but an important one. Certainly, developing good word processing skills will be a bonus for the individual for the rest of their life. If word processing is the individual's normal way of working, then they may also be able to do this in exams later.

Of course, the other benefit of using a computer is that presentation is improved and also the world of assistive technology opens up to the individual. This includes things like mind mapping, text reading and voice recognition software, along with a range of other supportive tools.

For many dyslexic adults many of the challenges that they experienced as children with literacy start to have far less impact when assistive technology is put to good use. It therefore makes sense to enable children to also have access to this sooner rather than later in order that they can prepare for the next part of their life, be that at college, at university or in work.

---

2   www.bdadyslexia.org.uk.

Encouraging writing at home

Where an individual is reluctant to write, the first step is to provide a clear purpose to the activity and a 'pay off' for the individual. Sadly, Christmas and birthdays only come around once a year, but writing a wish list of presents or even the activities they want to do that week is a great opportunity to practise writing.

As always, any practice is better than no practice; connecting to the interests and abilities of the individual is vital. For example, filling out forms to book activities is still writing, creating recipes is writing, social media posts to friends and family are still writing, and so on. Asking for help with writing shopping lists is effective, especially if they can add their own items. The bonus of these tasks is that they are short and manageable rather than formal and lengthy; they also have a clear purpose.

A handy hint here is to control the volume of the writing that is required. It is better to give a small piece of paper and have the child ask for more, than to give a large piece of paper that leaves them feeling overwhelmed. Likewise creating simple writing frames (e.g. phone message pads, pre-structured shopping lists) that provide starter sentences and vocabulary or provide a structure can help get the writing going.

One important word of caution here: as a parent try not to be judgemental. Remember the effort of writing and the 'risk' of negative judgements being made are significant. It is easy to undo a lot of your good work with an innocently made criticism, so try and avoid pointing out poor handwriting and weak spelling and value the effort that has gone in rather than judging the quality of the output. Confidence in writing is key to encouraging more writing to happen.

Spelling

Unfortunately, no chapter on literacy would be complete if it didn't at least touch upon spelling!

Most dyslexic individuals learn to read what they need to read when they need to read it, even if it takes longer for them to acquire these skills at the early stages, though they may not read for pleasure even as adults. Spelling challenges are, however, much more difficult to overcome. In many cases this is where assistive technology can really help.

Spelling is harder to do than reading. For reading at least you have the word on the page in front of you to decode, but for spelling you have to rely solely on the brain's ability to process accurately the sounds in the spoken words in the correct order and then accurately match those sounds to the right symbol (letter) and then remember them all, and then remember how to write those letters.

This is something that dyslexia most impacts upon. Phonological processing issues make it difficult to accurately identify and segment the sounds, and issues with short-term memory make them easily forgettable before you even get to matching them to the correct letters. Spelling is hard!

All of the work in the first section of this chapter on developing phonological awareness should really help with spelling and developing the ability to identify the individual sounds in words. Lots of practice will be required with matching these sounds to the correct letter.

A few other things that can help are:

◇ **Making good use of analogy**: In theory, if you can spell house you should be able to spell mouse, louse, spouse, etc. Dyslexic individuals may not notice the consistency in language and see no similarity in these words, instead thinking about a house as somewhere you live, a mouse as a small furry rodent, and a louse will result in some smelly shampoo and so on. Pointing out the consistent features in words can be helpful for spelling.

◇ **Mnemonics**: Some words are just tricky to spell and using mnemonics can help. They should, though, be 'owned' by the individual and practised frequently. Common ones are Big Elephants Can Always Use Small Exits (because) and Sally Ann Is Dancing (said) and Oh U Lucky Duck (-ould endings for could, would, should). Great care should be taken to not overload the individual with mnemonics, or you could end up with elephants dancing with lucky ducks! They help but should be used in moderation with the ultimate aim that the word can be spelt without having to rely on them.

◇ **Spelling rules**: A surprising amount of the English language is regular and follows rules and patterns. Whilst it is not a good approach to teach these in isolation, it can be helpful to point them out when they occur and provide additional hooks upon which to hang spelling knowledge. Many people do not know many spelling rules as they just pick this knowledge up through reading and writing experience. Because many dyslexic individuals do not read widely and write extensively, they can find it useful to have these rules and consistent patterns explicitly pointed out as and when they occur. There are several websites that will be able to provide these rules if you do not know them, and do not worry as very few people do actually know them all.

◇ **Suffixes, prefixes and syllables**: All of these have been covered in the reading section, but they can also help with spelling. These approaches enable the individual to break longer words down into bitesize chunks, that are often smaller and more regular, so spelling becomes a bit easier as the sounds match the letters in a more expected way.

Spelling tests

As a final parting point to this chapter, we do need to talk about spelling tests in school. These are often the stuff of nightmares for dyslexic children. They may put in large amounts of effort that is then not rewarded by the marks they achieve. They then get further demoralised by this failure.

An additional issue is often that the spellings learned do not then get transferred to their main writing activity. This could be because the spellings are filed in memory as something for that day and time, but not retrievable in different contexts.

If spelling tests must be given it is far more helpful for the individual to focus on particular personalised lists that make use of analogy, rather than random lists of words. It may be useful to discuss this in detail with your child's school to find a solution that builds confidence and is appropriately adapted to the needs of the individual child.

Concluding words

Literacy learning for many dyslexic children is particularly hard. The additional effort they have to put in may not yield immediate results. Any opportunity to make learning fun and game-based should be taken, and this also helps with facilitating the additional practice that might be required. Likewise, every opportunity to link this learning to areas of the child's particular interest will make the learning experience more rewarding for them.

This is an area where, as a parent, you need to have a close relationship with your child's teacher. If something really is not working, then discuss it with their teacher to see if there can be an alternative approach used that might be more effective.

Key takeaways

- Developing literacy in young people with dyslexia is a complex area and you should not feel like you need to be an expert – that is why schools exist. However, understanding the principles and some practical activities you can do with your child is really helpful.

- Phonological awareness is the starting point for all literacy learning.

- Reading requires more than just phonological awareness. Whilst this comes naturally to some children, young people with dyslexia are likely to need support with developing these skills.

- The reality is that for many dyslexic children, learning to be literate is very hard work. This can have a negative impact on your child's motivation to learn and on confidence and self-esteem. The key to success with supporting this area is to learn through fun and games, ideally using material that is of interest to your child.

References

Adams, M.J. (1998) *Phonemic Awareness in Young Children: A Classroom Curriculum*. Sydney: MacLennan & Petty.

Goswami, U. (2019) 'A neural oscillations perspective on phonological development and phonological processing in developmental dyslexia.' *Linguistic Compass 13*, 5, e12328. https://doi.org/10.1111/lnc3.12328.

Overy, K., Roderick, I., Fawcett, A.J. & Clarke, E.F. (2003) 'Dyslexia and music: Measuring musical timing skills. *Dyslexia 9*, 1, 18–36.

Further reading and resources

Books

Cowling, K. & Cowling, H. (1993) *Toe by Toe: A Highly Structured Multi-sensory Reading Manual for Teachers and Parents*. K & H Cowling.

Cowling, H. & Cowling, M. (2005) *The Hornet Literacy Primer*. H.J. Cowling.

King, H. & Wyatt, P. (1995) *Practice Punctuation: Book 1*. Penn: Hilda King Educational

King, H. & Wyatt, P. (1996) *Practice Punctuation: Book 2*. Penn: Hilda King Educational

Literacy for Life book series for acquiring reading and spelling skills. By Kathleen Paterson. Available at https://www.egon.co.uk/page/literacy-for-life.

New Reading and Thinking and *Reading for Meaning* series are available from Learning Materials at https://www.learningmaterials.co.uk.

Sandman-Hurley, K. (2019) *Dyslexia and Spelling: Making Sense of It All.* London: Jessica Kingsley Publishers.

Audio book resources

Bookshare – www.bookshare.org/cms/country/uk.
Calibre Audio – www.calibreaudio.org.uk.
Listening Books – www.listening-books.org.uk.

Websites and tools

Handwriting – https://nha-handwriting.org.uk.
Reader Pen – www.scanningpens.co.uk.
SEN Books – www.senbooks.co.uk.

CHAPTER 7

Why Organisational Skills Are Important for Young People with Dyslexia and How to Develop Them

BRITISH DYSLEXIA ASSOCIATION

Summary

◇ Why young people with dyslexia are likely to have issues with organisation.

◇ The principles of installing good organisational skills that last.

◇ Practical ideas for helping your child keep organised for school and home.

Being organised is a problem for many children, but for those who are dyslexic being organised can be particularly challenging. Issues with memory, combined with difficulties with sequencing can all lead to problems with organisation.

For the child this could mean turning up at school with the incorrect equipment, forgetting homework, and generally having a chaotic existence. This in turn can lead to frequent outbursts of frustration, as well as sanctions and detentions, not to mention dealing with frustration from teachers who once again are faced with a child minus PE kit, reading book, homework, etc.

Many parents will experience the morning chaos of the lost shoes, books, bags or kit, not to mention the last-minute requests for some obscure vital item for that school project that you knew nothing about up until that moment.

In other words, it can lead to a breakdown in the relationship between teacher and learner or indeed parent and child. Frustration builds on all sides.

Where do the difficulties start?

It is important to remember that for individuals who are dyslexic being disorganised is not always their fault. That does not mean that they cannot learn to become organised but it does mean they may need to be taught the skills and strategies that are required to be able to undertake certain tasks systematically and that 'safety nets' are in place for when an individual is having a 'bad day'.

Memory issues

Many individuals who are dyslexic have weaker short-term and working memory. Put simply, short-term memory is the ability to remember a piece of information for a short period of time and then recount it, usually in the same form.

A dyslexic individual may struggle to remember more than two or three pieces of information at any one time. If the number of pieces of information exceeds this amount, then they will simply not be processed. Another way to think of it is as a shelf. If the items placed on the shelf exceed the space available, then something will drop off. It is important to note that this is different from something that we forget but then remember when prompted. In the case of overload for a dyslexic person, some items did not make it onto the memory shelf, so there is no recollection of them. This again can lead to great frustration and potential conflict as the individual with the weak short-term memory may well deny all knowledge of ever being given that piece of information and this can therefore lead to many fruitless accusations followed by vehement denials. The simple answer is if the information never made it onto the memory shelf, for the dyslexic individual it never existed.

Working memory is, in simple terms, the part of memory that is used for sorting, filing and retrieving information. It allows us to store information in the correct place and then retrieve it for future use.

Getting started

Strange as it may seem, the best people to work out organisation strategies are the people who do not yet have them – the individuals themselves. If any sort of support in this area is going to be effective the individual must buy into it.

Broaching the subject with the individual is, however, likely to be a bit tricky, as it may well be perceived as criticism. It is important to pick your time carefully. This means that during a major disorganisation crisis is probably not a good time. Select a time when things are calm.

Human beings have a great need to feel in control. If you are disorganised, you rarely feel in control. Instead, it feels like you lurch from one surprise crisis to another, that horrible drowning feeling when we feel overwhelmed. Hopefully developing organisational strategies will help to remove these feelings.

The individual must own the process and the strategies that they use must be their own. Trying to inflict your methods on someone else whose brain does not operate in the same way as yours is unlikely to be successful. Therefore, the first part of the process must be to listen to what the individual has to say. What is their perception of their own organisational skills?

The role of the support provider

⬧ Work collaboratively with the individual; make suggestions but do not dictate.

⬧ Identify a range of different strategies that might be helpful, but do not get offended if these are rejected; allowing the individual personal choice and control is important within this process.

⬧ Explore each suggested approach in detail with the individual and discuss its merits and pitfalls, but try not to make it a 'sales pitch' for the one that you think is best.

⬧ Provide lots of opportunities for the individual to consider what they think might work and also discuss why this is the case.

- ◇ Identify and discuss any existing strategies, even if they may not in fact be helping, but do consider and talk these through to see if the current strategies can be developed/honed to meet the individual's needs.

- ◇ Dyslexic individuals need to have lots of opportunities to practise new learning and techniques so there needs to be time for this. Trying to develop organisational strategies in a crisis is unlikely to be successful.

- ◇ Very few things in life are perfect at first attempt. Therefore, we need to make sure that we check in with the individual and review what is working/not working and how things could be improved. It is also important to praise the positive improvements that have happened.

- ◇ Recognise that things are unlikely to always work 100 per cent of the time and therefore we need to make sure that there are safety nets in place, particularly for the really important things.

- ◇ Provide lots of encouragement; implementing new strategies will feel more arduous at first than just muddling along as before.

- ◇ Be aware that your role is not to do it for them or to nag them to do it for themselves. As a parent or carer, frankly sometimes it probably is just easier to do it yourself for the individual, but try not to if you possibly can. As for nagging, well we are only human, but try to avoid it if at all possible!

The following questions should start to provide some focus. They should also start to bring some of the most common barriers to being organised out into the open so they can be addressed directly.

Why am I doing this task?

Responses such as 'because I was told to' or 'because I have to' may be honest, but they are not very motivational. It sometimes helps to look at the bigger picture. For example, this task will help me to stop being shouted at in the morning or completing this task will allow me to get on and do the things I want to do rather than the things I have to do.

Dealing with something rather than putting it off usually also makes the individual feel better in the sense that they have actually done something rather than spent effort on avoiding the task. Task avoidance can be very exhausting!

What's in it for me?

Most people are reward driven; in order to do something that we find hard there has to be a pay off or a benefit of some kind. Sometimes these rewards, though, seem too distant.

Rewards that are immediate are much more effective, for example, if I do this now it will give me free time tomorrow to do something I want to do, or completing this work now means I can have an extra ten minutes in bed tomorrow.

What do I want to achieve?

Goal setting is an important part of any organisational process. It gives us something to aim for and when that goal is achieved, we know that the task is finished. The problem with goals is that they have to be achievable; if not, we soon become disheartened and give up. It is therefore much better to have different sets of goals to suit different circumstances.

By breaking a task down into manageable goals, we can achieve a larger outcome in smaller, much more achievable steps. For example, a parent might say, 'I want you to complete your homework before you can watch TV.' Immediately the child knows that this is a massive task and effectively it will be a long time before they can watch TV. The child ends up overwhelmed and demotivated before they start.

An alternative might be to review what homework needs to be done and then to break it down into bursts of ten minutes with ten-minute TV breaks in between.

Reviewing progress is important, so we can see that we have completed something and that we are progressing.

How could I make this task more interesting?

Let us be honest, some tasks are just plain boring, so we also need to think of ways of making some things more interesting – depending on the task there are often ways to bring something to life and reduce the boredom factor.

Am I taking this one step at a time? Can I break this task down into manageable steps?

Breaking a large task into manageable steps and goals makes it achievable. Perhaps the easiest way to tackle this is to write down or draw a mind map of everything that needs to be done or a to-do list. In order to be effective absolutely everything needs to be included. This approach also means that sometimes some tasks may overlap, so doing one thing resolves something else. It is helpful to prioritise tasks. Colour coding to order tasks into what needs to be done first, second, third and so on can be a useful approach.

Are my goals realistic with the time frame I have?

Now that the big task has been broken down into smaller steps, we need to attach a notional idea of how long each of these individual steps will take. At this point it is very important to be honest and realistic. We all tend to underestimate how long a particular task will take. In real life very few things are actually achieved in the often quoted two or five minutes.

Within this process there also needs to be break and contingency time. Contingency time is basically to allow for times when something has gone a bit astray and taken longer than expected. If such time is built in, then it reduces stress levels because we know there will be time to complete that activity later on or, if needed, we can take longer on it in the knowledge that we can catch up with other things later.

Am I relaxing and taking breaks?

Relaxation and breaks actually make us more effective. Break times should, however, be time-limited and scheduled.

Am I finding excuses?

We can often put more energy into thinking up reasons, excuses, for not doing something than it would take to actually do the thing.

When supporting an individual who has an excuse to cover every occasion, it is very important to get these out into the open and deal with them directly. This can be achieved by asking them to think of every excuse they have ever used to avoid doing something. Then ask them to imagine that they were the person on the receiving end of the excuses and to come up with solutions to them.

Excuse	Potential solution
I'm tired	Take a five-minute break
I can't be bothered	Set achievable goals, focus on the rewards
I don't understand it	Find someone to explain it or research it
It's boring	Think of three ways you could make it interesting

Do I have the right equipment?

There is nothing worse than starting a task only to find that, although you have found the motivation to do it, you do not have the right equipment. It is worth making a list of everything that you are likely to need before you start and then taking an inventory of whether or not it is available.

Am I likely to be interrupted? Am I aware of my distractions and can I deal with them?

Where an individual is undertaking work that requires high levels of concentration, it is important to identify potential sources of interruption and reduce them where possible. For example, turning the ring tone down on a phone and switching off notifications can prevent interruptions. This is about thinking of as many potential interruptions as possible and either ensuring that they are removed before work starts or having in place a strategy to reduce them.

Most people have certain things that they find particularly distracting. In order to work effectively, it is important to recognise what these are and where possible deal with them or, better still, build them into the organised work approach so that they are used effectively as rewards when work has been achieved.

Do I work well at this time of day?

Most people have certain times of day when they work most effectively. It is a good idea to try whenever possible to utilise the rhythm of someone's natural peaks and troughs in energy. If an individual is a morning person, then work that is more challenging should be done during this time. If the individual takes a while to get warmed up, then it is probably better to leave harder tasks until later in the day.

Is the task a priority or should I be doing something else?

Hopefully by breaking down and analysing the tasks that need to be done a series of priorities will have arisen, depending on things like deadlines, etc. For many individuals working out priorities can be challenging, especially when it all looks like it all needed doing yesterday. This is a skill that needs to be learnt and practised to avoid living in a state of permanent crisis management. A good question to ask is, 'What will happen if this task does not get done?' Hard tasks do not go away, they just cause anxiety!

Organisational preferences

The way that people like to be organised varies from one person to another. Anyone who has visited someone else's house will have noticed the different ways that people like to exist and how they order their lives. From the completely minimalist approach with everything lined up in an orderly sequence through to the seemingly chaotic, we all like to make our environments our own.

Children are no different and often this can indicate a particular organisational preference. Yes, even that teenage bedroom that resembles a cave is probably indicative of an organisational style, however well it might be hidden! It can, therefore, be useful as a parent to take a step back from tidying the bedroom of your child and actually take a bit of a deeper look to see if you can identify any particular consistencies in the way that they have organised their space.

Some individuals like to have everything in view because if they cannot easily see it, it does not exist for them! Therefore, if important things are put away and are out of sight they may well be lost and take more time to find. This can create a seemingly chaotic environment with lots of piles of seemingly irrelevant things. But quite possibly each of those items is in fact some form of memory trigger. Colour, pictures and images can be effective tools to help with organisation for this type of organisational preference, as is open fronted shelving.

When reviewing your child's room, you may find that you can see that they like to put things into some sort of sequential order, be it size or colour or category. Although their ordering may not be the same as your own, it is there, and it is important that they are able to use tools and approaches that allow them to do this.

Finally, there are those individuals who like to immerse themselves in their environment. They need to be comfortable in their environment and with any tools that they are going to use. Everything needs to be within easy reach, so getting items out of drawers or cupboards or storage systems just is not going to work. Once we have got some idea of the individual's organisational preferences, we can start to tailor our suggestions and approaches so that they are more likely to appeal to these preferences.

The school bag

It is a brave parent indeed that ventures into their child's school bag, but unfortunately this must be done. If it is chaotic and full of random pieces of paper (usually important notes home from three weeks ago) and rubbish, then this an area that needs work.

For those for whom comfort is everything, they will want

a bag to feel good when they are carrying it and one that is easy to open. Others who prefer a more ordered approach may well do better with a bag that has lots of individual pockets that can be used for specific items. Those with a visual preference may like a bag that opens up really wide so that they can see everything inside it easily.

Ring binders and folders

There are numerous types of ring binders available, but the ones with two rings avoid wasting time trying to find a hole punch for more holes. In the back it is always worth putting in a good supply of plastic 'punched pockets', as these will be important to store any loose bits of paper that might be collected throughout the day and can then be filed easily at the end of the day. Using different coloured or labelled by subject punched pockets can be useful to allow the individual to quickly identify which loose paper goes where. Subject dividers are also important so that the individual can quickly find the section that they need. It is also useful to include a small pencil case that can be hole punched and secured within the binder to hold spare pens, pencils, highlighters and so on, for those days when individuals have forgotten their pen or other necessary equipment.

Ring binders should be labelled on the spine, front and also on the back so whichever way round they might be they are easy to identify.

Some individuals may prefer a separate ring binder for each subject. Using different colours here can be useful as it means that the folder can be found quickly and easily. Others may well find a single folder with large dividers for each section, topic or work task easier to manage as this keeps everything in one accessible place.

Use plastic boxes to file full ring binders and again label them clearly, ideally one box per subject. If the files are placed in the box with spine facing up, they will be easy to find later for revision purposes. It is also useful as an additional referencing system to either add dates to the spine or number them.

In and out trays

This is basically simply a system of managing the work that has not yet been dealt with by filing and adding it to the schedule. It is not simply a dumping ground for things that the individual does not know what to do with.

When information is placed in any of the trays it is useful to date each piece as this gives an idea of when something arrived. Therefore, if something is not dealt with it gives an idea of the length of time it has been sitting there; date stamps are really helpful for dyslexic children.

An alternative to the in and out trays that can be particularly effective for young children is to use a two-pocket bi-folding folder – the left-hand pocket is clearly labelled 'take home', the right-hand pocket is clearly labelled 'take to school'.

Note and exercise books

Some individuals may prefer to or may have to use note-books. These can be a particular problem for learners who are dyslexic. Often the paper within these is of a poor quality and what is written on one side of a page tends to distort the writing on the other side of the page; they are not usually very robust so tend to fall apart very quickly. Once such a book is full it tends to disappear into a black hole never to be seen again, which can cause big problems when the information contained within it is required for revision.

It is possible to recover such exercise books and add a cardboard insert under the cover to help make them sturdier. If this is done, then specific coverings can be used for specific subjects, making it easier to quickly recognise the correct book for the correct subject rather than ending up in a biology class looking at a history exercise book.

Some teenagers may not want their equipment to stand out so marking books discreetly with some form of colour coding can be effective. It is worthwhile informing the subject teachers of these sorts of actions, otherwise the child may get into trouble for defacing their books.

Once full, an exercise book should be stored in a box that is specific for that subject.

If the child receives handouts during the course of a lesson it is important that these are attached firmly into the exercise book. It may therefore be necessary to provide the child with either a stapler or sticky tape, but always check school policy to see if they are allowed to have these items.

With your child, have a look at a stationery catalogue and discuss the various available options of ring binders, notebooks, filing and storage options. Try and identify what they feel might work well for them. Make sure they can explain to you why they think the ones they like will work, ensuring that decisions are not based on other, more personal, preferences that have nothing to do with being organised!

Being organised between home and school in the ideal world!

The title here says it all. The following is an ideal scenario of what we might like to happen and one that we can certainly try to achieve, but remember, any small step is better than nothing!

Children have to take work home for completion in the form of homework. Being in transit frequently poses a lot of issues for a dyslexic individual who struggles with personal organisation. It becomes a lot easier to lose items along the way and indeed by the time individuals have gone from one location to another they have often forgotten what they need to do. Therefore, strategies need to be in place.

In simple terms, any work that is going to be done away from school needs to be recorded. It then needs to be collected, stored in one place, transported, unpacked, sorted, completed, recorded, stored, and transported back. There is so much that can go wrong in that process.

Recording homework

Most children at school are given a planner, yet many of our dyslexic children struggle to use a planner. Therefore, we may need to find an alternative to this.

For younger children, the volume of work coming home should fit into a bi-folding folder, marked 'home' and 'school'.

If a diary or planner is used this should be encouraged, but do not be too disappointed if this system does not work well for the dyslexic child. It is helpful to put a large paperclip or bulldog clip on the page that relates to the current day to make it easier to find the right page when using it throughout the day. Alternatively, a simple 'home' to-do list to jot things down on as they occur can be effective. It is easy to develop a template document of this that can be printed out as needed.

An alternative strategy might be to use sticky notes. As a piece of work is given or identified throughout the day the individual writes it on sticky notes. The problem with these notes is that they are small and easily get lost. In order to deal with this, the individual could use a wallet (like the ones used for credit cards) and place each sticky note into the wallet once they have jotted down the work that is required

For some dyslexic learners, the act of writing down homework and assignments that are put on the board in the last 30 seconds of a lesson is a nightmare. This may mean that discussions need to be had with the teacher to ensure that homework is given at the beginning of the lesson, or at the very least at a time when the individual has enough time left in the lesson to record it.

For older learners an alternative to writing it down is to record it in some other form, e.g. if it is written on the board to take a photo of it with a mobile phone or to use a voice recording facility on a phone where they can dictate the task themselves. This is a good strategy, as any additional comments or parameters may be fresh in their mind. If using the voice recording option, it is important that they also state the date upon which the recording was made and any deadlines for completion for future reference. Lots of smartphones have a notes facility and this is useful, particularly when synched to a calendar or computer.

Collecting homework

Once the work has been recorded, all of the various bits need to be collected. Again, the bi-folding folder does this. If this is not being used, then the individual should review briefly any sticky notes, lists, photos, or voice recordings to ensure that they have what they need before leaving. If their bag has different compartments in it, one of these can be designated 'work for taking home'; if not then use a plastic wallet.

Unpacking homework

Once at home then the work needs to be unpacked. It is probably better to unpack everything as it prevents tasks being forgotten if they have gravitated to the bottom of the bag. Double check against the planner, sticky notes, photos or recordings that everything is there that should be there.

Sorting homework

Sorting is an important activity because often there will be work that needs doing immediately as well as work that has a longer deadline. Therefore, the work needs to be prioritised and categorised. It is quite useful at this point to colour code items, for example, red for things that need doing urgently, green for things that need doing in a couple of days, blue for things to do if there is enough time that day.

If using the sticky notes strategy, then these notes should be stuck onto an academic year wall planner that has the days of the week on it. It is then easy to see what work needs to be done and when. Where an individual has regular weekly activities such as clubs, these can be included on the wall planner. This makes it easy to see when life is going to get busy, so work can be scheduled to be done on days when things are a little less pressured.

Completing homework

Once all the work is sorted then it can be completed. It is useful to keep a checklist to hand when doing this as it provides great satisfaction to tick things off as each is done. Sometimes with a dyslexic child it is important for the parent to set the parameters of the work, particularly where the volume of homework seems inappropriate for the child. This is useful information to take back into school and use to negotiate with teachers on what is an appropriate amount of work to be done.

Recording and storing completed homework

For this purpose, it is useful to have a selection of boxes, trays, or a similar system marked with each day of the week. Each piece of completed work is placed in the place that corresponds with the day that it is required. The individual then just has to check the relevant place and collect the contents or place in folders if done online.

Transporting homework back to school

Completed work can then be placed in the individual's bag. For those individuals that have great difficulty in remembering to take their bag with them as they leave, a good strategy is to place a large notice somewhere where it will be the last thing they see before leaving home such as on the back of the door. This notice should be bold and stand out and also potentially have a final checklist of everything they need to take on it.

A word about homework and college assignments safety nets

All of the above is helpful but we also have to be realistic and accept that despite all of these best efforts sometimes things will go wrong. We therefore need to ensure that there are some safety nets in place. These could be:

- ◇ Use a classroom buddy or friend to check they have got the correct work and information.

- ◇ Check in with the teacher(s) regularly.

- ◇ Check the school website or eLearning platform regularly for any important updates.

By implementing some of these techniques and strategies, it is hoped that your child will become slightly better organised and you will be able to enjoy a slightly less manic morning.

☙ Key takeaways

- A young person with dyslexia is very likely to have issues with organisation due to challenges with short-term memory; organisation skills are important for school and life.

- It is important to understand how your child organises themselves and supports themselves to develop strategies that work for them. Do not force strategies upon them.

- To succeed with developing organisational skills for your dyslexic child, follow these top tips:

  › Keep any strategies simple – anything over complicated is likely to fail and adds to the memory burden of trying to remember it.

  › Develop routines – same thing, same time, each day. Routine is your best friend.

  › Have a place for everything and try to put everything in this place.

  › Make good use of to-do lists.

  › Do not expect perfection – some chaos is likely and to be expected with a dyslexic child!

  › Review and evaluate constantly – if something is not working after a decent attempt at it, try something else.

CHAPTER 8

The Value of Study Skills for Dyslexic Learners and How to Acquire Them

BRITISH DYSLEXIA ASSOCIATION

Summary

◇ What study skills are and why they are particularly important for dyslexic learners.

◇ Common study challenges faced by young people with dyslexia.

◇ Essential study skills and how to acquire them.

A great deal is often said about study skills, but what in fact are they?

Whilst natural aptitude, passion for the subject and hard work are important, study (accessing information and demonstrating understanding through a task such as an essay) involves specific skills. These skills are learnt, like any others. For dyslexic learners, it is particularly important to develop good study skills as the challenges dyslexia presents can create more barriers to studying.

It will not matter how good an individual is at study skills, if they know nothing about the subject, they are unlikely to pass the exam at the end of the course! Having said that, being able to think about their knowledge effectively, apply the knowledge appropriately, and communicate that knowledge to others efficiently will mean that success is more likely. Knowledge and study skills are intrinsically linked.

Study skills fall into a number of areas, from effective reading and researching through to participation in lessons and applying this information to assignments or tasks. For many dyslexic individuals, the burden of trying to learn in an environment that does not work well for them anyway, where they are often just trying to keep up, means that they do not often get the head space or time to even consider how to learn more effectively. Yet it is for these learners that techniques that act as shortcuts and aid efficiency are likely to have the greatest impact.

The caveat here is that each individual will be different, and their individual preferences should be accounted for; what works for one person may not work for another. Likewise, much will depend on the subject being studied and the level of that study.

The most important stage in the process when starting to study or work on an assignment is to clarify exactly what is required. This may seem an obvious first step but sometimes the way that an assignment brief has been written may be perfectly clear to the tutor, but not at all clear to the student.

Break down the question

Using the following approach to break down the question can assist the student with identifying what is required.

It should be stressed though that, if at any time the student is unclear about what exactly they are supposed to be doing then their first port of call should always be the tutor or lecturer that has set the assignment. This can save a lot of time and potential distress in the future.

⬦ **Topic area/subject matter**: Underline words that indicate subject matter.

⬦ **Limiting words, aspect and focus**: Highlight the words that control the discussion areas of the topic.

⬦ **Directive or instruction**: Highlight the words that direct approach, purpose and provide marking criteria.

Plan the attack

Look at when the assignment is due in and then work backwards from this point. It may be that the deadline seems a long way in the future, but it is surprising how quickly time goes by and what seems like a long time can suddenly become a very tight, if not impossible deadline.

Frequently, dyslexic individuals will underestimate how long reading, researching, drafting and checking will take, so being generous with the time that is scheduled is the best approach. Also, contingency time should be built in as inevitably other things will come along that will throw even the best laid plan out of whack. The saying 'If you fail to plan, you are planning to fail!' is potentially true in this case.

Individuals may need some support to do this entirely linear and sequential task, particularly as effectively they will be working backwards from the completion or submission date to the present. This type of task can be particularly challenging for a dyslexic individual. Resources such as wall planners can be exceptionally useful for this activity and are a visual reminder for the individual. Different subjects can be colour coded and mapped onto the chart, so it provides an at a glance overview of what an individual has got on, what is in the pipeline and where any pinch points are likely to be.

Breaking a long timeline into shorter achievable tasks, goals or outcomes is also far more effective and less overwhelming. This allows the individual to chart their progress effectively and they can recognise their progress more easily. Setting alarms and reminders on calendars can be really helpful to keep the individual on track.

Encouraging frequent reviews and adapting the timeline also means that the individual can adapt to any changing priorities and demands. Also, do not forget to build in down time and fun activities. These are just as important as work and in fact can lead to greater productivity.

Double check and then check again the guidance for the assignment

There is nothing worse than putting loads of effort and time into a piece of work only to find out later that what you have done does not in fact answer the question. Dyslexic individuals can easily get distracted by interesting pieces of information or simply go off track; they are often great explorers of information. Make sure of what the parameters are with the piece of work – is there a word limit or marking scheme that might suggest where effort is best focused? If the individual is in any doubt about the guidance associated with the assignment they should go back to the tutor and ask for clarification. This can save a lot of wasted effort in the long run.

It can also be really helpful to write the assignment title onto a large piece of paper and pin it up in front of where the individual will be working. In this way they can frequently look at it and remember what is being asked and so stay on track and focused.

Additionally, if they are working on something else and a piece of information or inspiration comes to them about that assignment, they can quickly make a note of it on the piece of paper pinned up in front of them so that they don't forget it later.

Dyslexic individuals are sometimes described as 'good procrastinators', i.e. they take their time to incubate the best solutions. Using this strategy allows the brain to consider the question during other activity. It also takes account of potential memory challenges and facilitates the capture of that thought before it is forgotten.

Most tutors do not set pieces of work just to torture their students, so it can be helpful to also think about how and why this piece of work might have been set. The student might like to consider what they have been working on in taught sessions. Did there seem to be a particular focus? Is the tutor particularly attached to a subject, theory or concept? If so, it is probably best to ensure that this is included. How does this assignment relate to the topic being studied as a whole? Many dyslexic individuals are 'big picture' thinkers and considering a piece of work in this holistic way can help with recognising its relevance and how it will fit within the broader subject being studied.

How should the student present the work?

Sometimes when working on an assignment there will be parameters around how the piece of work should be structured, for example, is it a formal essay, can bullet points be used, is it a report format, what are the criteria for referencing and so on?

A badly presented piece of work or a piece of work that does not follow the required conventions may well lose marks regardless of how excellent the content is. This should be avoided if at all possible. It is particularly frustrating when the content of a piece of work is excellent but appropriate presentation conventions have not been followed.

Most schools, colleges or universities will have guidance on referencing and presentation and the dyslexic student should make a careful note of these. It can be useful to create a checklist for items such as inclusion of a front sheet, student number, referencing style and so on to use as a final review document before handing the work in. Again, there is nothing quite as frustrating as either having a piece of work rejected because presentation conventions have not been met or losing valuable marks unnecessarily.

An aspect that dyslexic students may struggle with is the format of certain types of documents, particularly if they do not read extensively. For example, if being asked to write a report, a formal essay, a synopsis, summary or literature review, lack of reading experience can trip dyslexic individuals up. If you do not know what the writing conventions are for these types of documents, it is hard to know what the structure of them is and what they should look like.

The best way of tackling this is to find examples of similar documents. If in any doubt, clarification should be sought from the tutor or learning support service. This is not a sign of weakness. This is just a common-sense approach to prevent unnecessary errors.

Stand back and take in the view

When looking at an assignment it is easy for a dyslexic individual to feel daunted and overwhelmed; the planning process and setting a timeline with smaller achievable goals should help with this, but even so there can be the 'I know nothing about this topic' feeling. This in turn leads to the individual feeling overwhelmed by the scale of the task and potentially becoming paralysed into inaction.

It can be helpful here, in order to deal with these 'I can't' feelings, to try very quickly to brainstorm what they already know about this subject or related subjects. Often it is surprising what we do know – we have just forgotten we knew it! This is a good way to take positive action to prevent this thinking paralysis and feeling overwhelmed.

The other reason for doing this is that quite possibly there will be some research involved in completing the assignment, even if just reviewing course or class notes. There is little point spending time researching or reading about the areas of the topic that are already known. There might be a need to check facts and refresh, but there is not much point wasting precious effort on existing knowledge. This effort is better spent on exploring other areas where the knowledge is lacking.

Finding the information

There are numerous sources of information and for the dyslexic student this in itself can be overwhelming. Many courses of study will have a reading list and sometimes this is so huge that realistically no student is ever going to manage to read every item. For dyslexic students, often the simple fact of having a reading list, whilst helpful, can add to feelings of anxiety and inadequacy. They may labour under the notion that all the other students are reading every item on that list, though this is highly improbable.

A good approach here is to talk to the tutor and ask them which texts they would most recommend. This may shorten the list quite considerably. Alternatively, talk to other students and see what they have found to be most useful; even better, talk to other students who have completed that course or module successfully.

The traditional approach of going to the college or university library is still a good one. Librarians are usually incredibly helpful and may even be able to provide an insight into what are the most useful texts based on popularity. Learning to use effectively the cataloguing system is also likely to save time in the long run. Making friends with the librarian is a good tactic!

If using library resources, it should be remembered that core texts (or the most useful ones) are likely to be popular with other students; they may need to be reserved in advance and have a time restriction on them for how long they can be borrowed. Often a dyslexic student can have an extension on the loan period to take account of the additional time it might take them to read them, so it is always worth asking if this is possible.

Libraries also usually have a good stock of academic papers, or journals. For those studying in higher education these are vital. These can be particularly daunting for dyslexic students. A handy hint here is to find the key researchers on the topic in question; these are often the most prolific writers and will be cited by others frequently.

Most articles in journals have an abstract and these can prove to be extremely useful in identifying which articles are most relevant to the research. In addition, sometimes reading the abstract will yield the information required without reading the full article. This is not cheating!

There is an endless supply of information online, which can be overwhelming. For dyslexic individuals, researching online is often far easier than using books and libraries, particularly if they have text reading software available to them.

There is, though, a need to be careful about what information is used. The type of website that comes up from a search is often a good clue. The more academic ones tend to have a more traditional feel to them. Also it is important to check out whether or not the material is from a reliable source, such as a known publisher or university, rather than if it can be generated by any site user.

It can be helpful for a dyslexic student to learn how to use a search engine effectively. The way that words or phrases are put into a search engine will either narrow or broaden the number of results.

Getting a huge number of results when looking for something on the internet can be completely overwhelming for a dyslexic student. Not knowing what to look at and having to trawl through lots of content that is not relevant is both time consuming and offers too much opportunity for distraction and to stray away from the actual task. Using quotation marks around a phrase will narrow the search by making the search engine look for only the whole phrase, for example 'study skills'. Otherwise it will look for any pages where those same words come up individually in the page or in a different order, i.e. the page could mention 'study' somewhere and 'skills' elsewhere, but not be relevant to the topic you're looking for: information on 'study skills'.

Using a minus sign in front of words will cause a search engine to not include those words in the results, which is useful for excluding words that are distracting the search engine from the topic you are trying to find.

There are numerous online guides and videos that can explain how to use a search engine effectively and it is well worth honing these skills to narrow down results and make online searches more effective.

Whatever research method is used, one aspect that is vital is that the student makes a note of what the source is, the title of the book or journal, the names and initials of the authors, and the date it was published. Any referencing guidelines, such as using the Harvard referencing system, should be applied. There are ways of doing this electronically that can really help with referencing such as 'Cite This For Me' or 'MyBib'.

Selecting the information

Many dyslexic individuals assume that everyone else reads everything that is written on the page. This is often not the case – just think about when a skilled reader picks up a magazine or newspaper or book.

A variety of approaches are used, first to identify the interesting or relevant pieces that are going to be read and then, often, the proficient reader will skim (eyes moving quickly over the page to gain a general meaning) and scan (eyes seeking specific words or information) through the text to find the bits that are of particular interest or relevance.

As proficient readers we actually are also very selective readers.

◇ Initially we may look at the picture or image on the front of the book or magazine. If this draws our attention or appeals to our interest, we may continue to delve a little deeper.

◇ If we decide that the reading material looks interesting, we may flick through the whole thing to see whether or not it is of more interest, usually by glancing at pictures, images, or chapter or article headings. If it is not of interest, we will put it down and walk away.

◇ If the reading material looks of interest, we may then look a bit deeper, maybe looking at the introduction to articles or chapters, the contents list, etc.

◇ We may decide to scan through the text either for particular things of interest or for information.

◇ Pictures and diagrams can be particularly useful to capture our attention and provide a useful visual aid to help with understanding the content (as well as breaking up dense text, making it appear more accessible).

◇ Finally, after this process we may actually read the text in more detail.

Understanding this process and encouraging a learner who is dyslexic to use this approach can make them far more efficient in their choice of reading material. Rather than trying to read material that doesn't meet their needs, we need to encourage them to be more selective so that when they do invest the time and energy into actually reading something in detail they are getting the most out of that experience rather than battling away at something that doesn't meet their needs.

Individuals will need lots of practice with the above strategy and access to a variety of texts to hone these skills. Using a checklist to remind them of the approach can also be useful.

These strategies, when implemented appropriately, mean that an individual with fairly basic levels of reading skills can access text in a structured way and get the information that they need from that text without feeling totally overwhelmed by the reading task itself.

Reading the information

Possibly one of the most daunting tasks for a dyslexic individual is reading and researching effectively. Whilst many individuals will manage to read, they are likely to take a bit longer and quite often struggle with reading comprehension. This means that a piece of text may have to be read numerous times before any proper understanding of it is reached.

The further an individual progresses in education, the more the volume of independent reading is likely to increase. Therefore, developing strategies to tackle this area of challenge can be particularly helpful. On top of this, it is often not enough just to have read something; the individual is likely to have to be able to recall it at will and assimilate that information into other pieces of work.

Although some students may be genuinely interested in a topic and enjoy finding out as much as possible about it, more commonly a student will be carrying out research in order to complete a particular task or assignment. Even if the reading about the subject is being enjoyed, there is also the risk that the individual will disappear down a rabbit warren of interest and go off track from the purpose of the reading, which is to tackle the assignment.

Issues with reading for dyslexic students typically fall into some general categories; these are:

◇ **Quantity**: Just too much volume.

◇ **Difficulty**: The material is too complex especially where ideas or concepts need to be pulled out and then assimilated and put into the assignment.

◇ **Interest**: To be honest, some of the material that needs to be read may just be downright boring, so it is difficult to stay motivated and engaged.

There are some key 'active learning' strategies that can help the dyslexic student choose where to invest their effort and how to get the maximum value from this effort.

◇ Before starting to read the text, individuals need to think about what they already know about the subject and what they need to find out. This will allow them to skip what they already know and focus on filling in the gaps in their knowledge.

◇ Encourage individuals to have a quick flick through the text to see how accessible it feels – is it well spaced with lots of subheadings, sections and so on? This is likely to be far easier to navigate than pages of dense text.

◇ Look at the contents page – is what they are looking for listed in the contents? If it is, then there will likely be quite a lot of information about the thing they are looking for in one place. If it is just a few entries in an index then it likely to be something that is mentioned in passing, so may be worth coming back to, but most likely will not be covered in detail.

◇ When looking at a section encourage reading of introductions and conclusions first. This will identify what it is going to cover and what it concludes. They may get what they need just from this minimal amount of reading.

◇ Look at the first and last couple of sentences in paragraphs; again individuals might find this gives them the information that they need without reading the whole discussion in the paragraph.

◇ Skim through a piece of text and where there is new vocabulary or acronyms encourage individuals to make a note of these on postcards with a definition. These will act as useful revision tool later.

◇ Highlight any key words or phrases (if they own the text); use different colours to show differing points of view or points of varying importance.

◇ Make notes in the margins to summarise key points in their own words.

◇ Make summaries with a word limit of, say, ten to 15 words of key points.

◇ Write the key points on sticky notes and see if there are other ways in which the information could be presented.

◇ If the text is really hard going, try and find a more basic one or look online to establish a basic level of understanding first.

◇ Make an audio digital recording of the individual summarising what they have just read; again, this will be a useful revision tool.

◇ Suggest they pretend they are explaining it or teaching it to someone else.

◇ Devise some questions about the subject they are reading about and then try and answer them later; again, these may be a useful revision tool later.

◇ Encourage the individual to keep checking in with themselves to remember what they are looking for or trying to find out; they should keep checking back to the assignment task to ensure they are on track.

◇ Set a time limit; reading something hard is just hard! If the individual gets exhausted by the effort, they will not absorb what they are reading anyway so suggest a target of say no more than ten minutes, then have a break and do something else.

◇ Encourage the individual to make a mind map or draw a diagram or flow chart about the subject; again, this will provide a useful quick revision tool later.

Staring at a text for hours on end in the hope that something will go in is unlikely to be helpful. It may also be worthwhile watching a video online or reading something else or talking to friends about it; all of these approaches are valid and help to prevent the individual from feeling overwhelmed.

Getting information from classes and lectures

Traditional 'chalk and talk' approaches to teaching and learning are unlikely to be particularly accessible for dyslexic individuals. This is due to the challenges associated with having to multitask and process lots of auditory information, copying from a screen whilst simultaneously trying to take notes. That said, it is likely that they will encounter this and, as with many things, preparation is key to successful study if faced with these situations.

It is always worth asking the tutor for handouts of PowerPoints or any other information in advance of the actual teaching session. If the individual has this information in advance it enables them to preview the subjects that are likely to be covered in the taught session. This could be through:

◇ watching videos online

◇ checking any unfamiliar vocabulary so they do not spend unnecessary time trying to work out what the new and unfamiliar words are

◇ identifying any questions or areas they really do not understand

◇ identifying key points and setting up a note making

template[1] so class notes can be added in a structured way during the session

◇ listening in for key words, names, dates, terms and definitions during the session and if possible, highlighting these in some way

◇ if possible and if allowed, taking photographs of key diagrams of discussion notes that are captured on a flip chart or similar

◇ filing any notes immediately after the taught session and adding any further actions to their to-do list to be scheduled later

◇ comparing notes with other students to ensure that nothing has been missed can also be useful.

Making notes

Making notes is particularly challenging for dyslexic individuals. The difficulties dyslexic individuals experience with working memory, speed of processing, writing speed and confidence with spelling all work against them. They may find it hard to decide what to write down and where. Often, they lose the thread of what is being said. The skills involved in note taking and making are:

◇ understanding the language

---

1   A note making template is a predesigned framework that might include boxes that can be filled with content, such as date of session, topic title, key vocabulary, key questions, key references and names, summary of areas covered, areas to explore more, conclusions, further reading, assignment information and so on.

◇ selecting what is important

◇ organising the information gained

◇ reorganising that information and presenting it in a different way.

Lots of unpressurised practice using short talks or videos, or reduced texts will help individuals to learn and practise the skills required. Some useful strategies are:

◇ Make sure notes are not crowded on the page in case more information needs to be added later. Drawing margins, one on the left and one on the right can help to ensure that there is room for later additions.

◇ Using bullet points and colour can really help notes come to life. Adding a short summary of the key points at the end is an effective technique and useful for revision later.

◇ For revision purposes it is also often useful to make an audio file of the notes. Using a digital recording device or even a mobile phone means that these files can be uploaded onto a computer, and for revision the learner can listen to their notes whilst following through them in their written form. This reduces the additional processing burden caused by potential reading difficulties.

Although many learners may attempt to record lessons and lectures, writing up notes from these recordings can be very time consuming and tiring, though such recordings are a useful back-up.

Note making techniques include:

◇ **The 6 Ws**: Using the 6Ws can be helpful. These stand for **W**here, **W**hat, **W**hen, **W**ho, **W**hy, How. These questioning words can be written in boxes and act as a writing frame as well as ensuring that the basic facts of the information being given are captured.

◇ **Timeline**: This sort of approach is useful for learners who are more linear thinkers. This approach would be particularly useful for plotting a historical event, a scientific experiment, a piece of literature and so on.

◇ **Key words and pictures**: In this approach the learner's page is split in half. On one side they write one or two key words and on the other half a picture or symbol to go with that piece of information.

◇ **Diagrams**: These are similar to the writing frames, for example, a Venn diagram can be particularly useful for compare and contrast activities.

◇ **Mind or concept mapping**: These use a combination of key words, images and colour. Some learners find these useful whilst others may really struggle with them. There is lots of mind mapping software available.

◇ **Photographs**: Taking photos of key slides and the like from presentations or flip charts can be a useful 'quick capture' method. These can then be annotated.

Although making notes is likely to be particularly challenging for a dyslexic individual, developing this skill is really important. There is no right or wrong way and certainly one single approach will not suit all individuals. Whatever way an individual makes notes, the following are vitally important:

◇ Ensure that the individual files their notes in a safe and accessible place. Time must be allocated to filing and organising notes. The best notes in the world are not going to be much help if they cannot find them when they need them. (The bottom of a bag or boot of a car is not an appropriate filing system!)

◇ Notes must be reviewed frequently to ensure that the information stays fresh and at the front of the individual's memory. Using increasing time intervals between reviews is a useful strategy to ensure that they do not forget the information and that the information is easily accessible in memory.

◇ Ensure the individual recognises the difference between simply recognising the information (it simply looks familiar) and recollection (they actually remember the content of the information).

◇ Using the strategies for active learning will help to embed the information in memory and enable the individual to engage with the information.

𐑍 Key takeaways

– Study skills, like all skills, are learnt and dyslexia learners can develop them well with good support.

– Learning to study effectively by planning and engaging in the material being studied is likely to mean that the individual becomes more effective in their learning.

– Dyslexic individuals really do need to engage in active learning processes. They cannot rely on memory alone.

- Once they know the subject they are studying, they really know everything about the subject they are studying. The dyslexic brain is hard wired to be an explorer of information and the suggestions in this chapter will hopefully mean that these explorations can be put to good use and help the individual to achieve academically.

Resources

Organisation
> www.hottnotes.com
> www.zhornsoftware.co.uk/stickies
> www.portablefreeware.com/?id=1250&ts=1258712098.
File management – www.audacityteam.org.
Annotations – www.tracker-software.com/product/pdf-xchange-viewer.
Grammar checker – www.gingersoftware.com.
Windows built-in speech to text – www.nuance.com – or for wide range of languages – http://imtranslator.com.

CHAPTER 9

Working with Your Child's School

DR HELEN ROSS

Summary

◇ What support to expect from your child's school.

◇ Key questions to ask your child's school.

◇ How to build a good working relationship with your child's school.

◇ What to do if the relationship with your child's school breaks down.

Working with young people in schools is a privilege.

As professionals, we can make or break families' and young people's engagement with education, switching them on to a whole new world of opportunity or turning them off learning completely, undermining their whole educational experience.

Much is made within current English policy around the voices of young people and their families being central to support programmes for young people in schools. Therefore, it is vital that professionals and families work together, positively and productively to support our young people. Where a young person has dyslexia or other specific learning differences, ensuring that appropriate provision is in place for them can be problematic.

This chapter suggests some of the things parents should consider when engaging with their child's school. Different ways that initial contact might be made with schools are suggested, as are ways of ensuring appropriate support for their child is in place before they start at the school and maintaining a successful relationship with the school.

Two case studies will show how parent–school interactions can affect provision for young people with dyslexia, as well as suggestions for moving forward when relationships deteriorate between parents, carers and school staff.

Finally, this chapter will conclude with a list of further reading for more information about provision or young people with special educational needs.

'My child has dyslexia.' What can you do about it?

Deciding to have your child assessed for dyslexia may be something that you have debated for a long time, or it may be a relatively new decision. Wherever your family situation lies between those two standpoints, once you have a Diagnostic Assessment that confirms dyslexia, it is important that your child knows that they are still the same person and that they are still valued. The things that your child finds tricky and the things they excel at will remain the same. However, now they have an understanding of why some things can be difficult for them.

Lots can be done to support young people with dyslexia both at home and at school, ranging from relatively expensive measures to free ways of working. They key to all support is that young people are engaged in it and feel that their voices are heard in discussions between them, their parents, carers and school.

Making initial contact with school

When contacting a school, it can seem like an impenetrable fortress into whose walls you shall not pass! However, that might just be because the website is tricky rather than an indication about the school itself.

If you are at the point of wanting to speak to someone in the school, quite often the best way of engaging with them is to just phone the reception. School receptionists often have all the answers to queries, and if they don't know the answer to a question, it is highly likely that they will know who to ask. They will point you in the right direction of SENCOs (Special Educational Needs Coordinators), year tutors, form tutors and anyone else you may need to contact.

A new setting

If you are choosing a new education setting, be it a first-time primary or nursery school, a transitioning-to-secondary move or a progression to college, usually there comes a point to engage with the SENCO and their team.

How this happens and what form it takes will depend as much on the school as the phase of education that your child is at. There will likely be differences if they are starting a new setting midway through a Key Stage, versus if they are transitioning between settings at expected times.

For young people with dyslexia, it is important that their class teachers know that they have it, so that adjustments can be made to the delivery of lessons and so that specialised and/or focused intervention can be put in place to support them where appropriate.

Starting school

When your child starts a new school, there is no doubt that you will have questions and want to know about its inner workings.

Once you have made the formal selection for your child, or even if you are still unsure where you will choose for your child, it is important to talk to their SENCO and, if possible, to meet the team. There will be things you want to know about the room(s) your child will work in, how the day breaks down, and what other young people in that setting are like, amongst other things. To find some answers to these questions, it is useful to visit the setting with your child. They may also have similar questions to you and benefit from some time to find their own answers, to put their mind at ease before formally starting in a setting. If you can, try to spend a good amount of time in the setting, with your child. If there is a cohort of students starting at the same time (e.g. Year 6 into Year 7), it is likely that there will be a formal transition day.

Where your child starts a new setting independently, try to organise a day where they will have at least a morning or afternoon session in the classroom with their new peers and teacher(s). That way they can experience that setting first-hand. They will be able to report back to you on their day and you can compare experiences. It will also help you to join up dots of written policies versus what young people experience on the ground. Hopefully there won't be too much dot-joining to be done and it will all be straightforward and clear.

During your child's classroom taster session is the ideal time for you to talk with the SENCO and their team. Here are a few suggestions of questions to ask when you do meet the SENCO and their team:

- ◇ How are young people with dyslexia identified within this setting?

- ◇ How is students' progress monitored?

- ◇ What kind of support is there for young people with dyslexia? Can you show me any examples of the kind of differentiation that teachers do in their classroom?

- ◇ How are general class teaching assistants (not 1:1 named pupil support teaching assistants) usually deployed?

- ◇ If my child finds using assistive technology easier and this is their usual way of working, what measures are in place to ensure that they can continue to use this to access the curriculum?

- ◇ How often and how do you review interventions and support for young people with dyslexia?

- ◇ Which member of staff will undertake reviews of the support in place for, and the progress of, my child?

- ◇ What procedures are in place surrounding Exam Access

Arrangements and what type of arrangements are usually in place for young people with dyslexia?

◇ If we feel that support provision is not enough for our child, what are the local procedures for requesting an assessment for an EHCP and how many children have you applied for in this setting?

◇ If we need to contact you, what is the best way to do so? (This is important as it could be that the SENCO works across various schools and/or is not available for contact every day. You might decide that the manner or regularity of contact expected in this setting is not suitable for you as a family.)

Transitioning

If your child is transitioning from primary school to secondary school, information should be passed between the schools. That should mean that your child's new setting has all the relevant information about your child, their dyslexia and its effect on their learning, and how your child's needs are met in class.

When your child starts a new setting their 'data' may not have reached their class teachers yet. With this in mind, it is usually a good idea to contact the SENCO and discuss how your child is best supported with them. If they feel able or wish to, it can be productive and empowering for your child to be part of discussions surrounding provision to support them.

Most schools have 'one-page profiles' of young people with Special Educational Needs and Disabilities (SEND), which detail how they work, what they enjoy and what they don't like. It is good practice for young people to be consulted on the content of these profiles.

Support strategies

This is not an exhaustive list of strategies, so be mindful that your child may have different ways of working. However, this is a list of 'reasonable adjustments' that may be implemented relatively easily within schools (and are currently implemented in many schools) and so whichever ones apply should be in place for your child. Discussions with the school SENCO should ensure that they are in place. The list may also prompt discussions of new strategies to support your child.

- ◇ **Note taking**: Gap fill exercises to replace note taking; copies of notes provided to reduce copying burden; extra time to take written notes where necessary; use of alternative recording methods such as photographs where possible.

- ◇ **Giving and following instructions**: Provision of visual prompts for instructions; short, clear and concisely listed tasks; use of bullet points to sequence activities; opportunities to discuss instructions with others to check understanding; reminders/prompts to help them stay on task; extra time to process and understand instructions.

- ◇ **Activities**: Worksheets copied onto coloured paper; shorter exercises; clear, sans serif font for worksheets; multisensory activities such as access to manipulatives in maths; sandboxes to practise letter formation;

mini whiteboards to practise responses; extra time to undertake tasks.

◇ **Planning work**: Opportunities to discuss work before committing ideas to paper; use of planning strategies such as mini whiteboards, sticky notes, mind maps, bullet points before starting tasks; extra time to plan work; sentence starters as prompts for content; model answers; use of assistive technology to allow for visual or oral planning.

◇ **Producing work**: Extra time to produce written work; use of assistive technology, such as a laptop and/or speech-to-text software, to help them produce textual responses to tasks; access to alternative recording methods such as video to record responses to tasks; where possible, access to a scribe to support with writing tasks; specific focus for tasks such as only focusing on one spelling pattern, content rather than spelling, paragraphs rather than capital letters, etc; model answers/responses to tasks.

◇ **Reading**: Use of assistive technology where possible to support reading; access to a reader to help them decipher tasks or more challenging tasks; allow young people with dyslexia to volunteer responses rather than requiring their participation in whole-class reading activities.

For some young people with dyslexia, more specialised interventions to support literacy may be necessary in the short (or longer) term, so that they can access other areas of the curriculum. There are various forms these can take, and they vary across schools, depending on capacity, staffing and young people's needs. Here are a few support strategies that may be in place. The list is not exhaustive, and it is always worth talking with your child's setting if you feel that more specialist provision is needed.

◇ **Reduced timetable**: Young people with dyslexia may be excused from certain aspects of the curriculum. If their literacy in English is weak, there may be justification to request that they are excused from learning an additional language or a humanities subject, such as history. This will reduce their workload and provide time during their working day so that they can focus on other subjects. Not all schools can offer such an arrangement; however, it can prove very successful when carefully implemented.

◇ **Small-group or one-to-one intervention**: In primary schools particularly, if young people have difficulty with their phonics (a key feature of dyslexia) in Key Stage 1, they may receive support in small groups outside of the mainstream classroom. This is often a first level intervention, after which most young people cease to receive such provision. In secondary schools, similar interventions may take place in Key Stage 3 to support literacy. Where an EHCP is in place, one-to-one literacy support via a specialist teacher or teaching assistant may be funded. In secondary school, the likelihood of small-group intervention is considerably less than in primary school. It is more likely that teachers are expected to meet your child's needs in class through differentiated work and high-quality delivery. If you are concerned that this is not happening, you should talk with the school SENCO in the first instance.

Following a Diagnostic Assessment

Where a Diagnostic Assessment has taken place, either via a school or setting or if you have commissioned it privately, it is important to meet with the SENCO in your child's setting to discuss its implications. The questions to be asked usually will be like those posed were your child moving schools or transitioning Key Stages alongside their peers, for example:

- ◇ What support do you provide for children with dyslexia?

- ◇ Will my child be able to access the exam arrangements recommended in the report?

- ◇ Do you provide access to hardware and software?

- ◇ Will my child receive 1:1 specialist teacher tuition?

- ◇ How do you monitor progress?

- ◇ How do you know if any intervention my child accesses has worked?

While a Diagnostic Assessment may provide you (as a parent) with explanations of your child's difficulties, there may be a period of transition for your child while they process and try to understand what it means for them to be dyslexic. Discussion of this with the SENCO can be important, as they likely have experience in supporting young people with dyslexia both academically and pastorally.

An important consideration is that much provision for young people is 'needs' based rather than as a result of a diagnosis alone. Thus, where your school has referred your child for a Diagnostic Assessment, it is likely that they are aware of their dyslexic tendencies and are making reasonable adjustments for them in class, alongside ensuring that teaching is suitable and of a high standard.

A Diagnostic Assessment may not automatically mean that provision for your child changes or that they receive small-group interventions. The type and level of provision should depend purely on your child's needs.

However, there are many other factors which are at play and may affect the setting's capacity to support young people with dyslexia. In any case, however, a positive and productive working relationship with your child's setting facilitates implementation of support.

CASE STUDY ONE – NIAMH

Niamh was an able student in Year 12 at a small independent school. Having achieved high grades in her sciences at GCSE, she embarked on physics A Level and enjoyed the subject. She had positive relationships with members of staff, and her family was highly engaged with school life.

However, she began noticing that she found processing mathematical concepts within physics very difficult. Decoding worded questions and linking to mathematical equations to understand the processes to be used was disproportionately difficult.

After a discussion with her parents and teachers, she was assessed to see whether she had an underlying specific learning difference. The Diagnostic Assessment revealed Niamh's relative weaknesses in phonological and visual processing, which impeded her ability to access the curriculum.

Following her Diagnostic Assessment, a learning profile was drawn up in consultation with her parents, Niamh herself and the teachers working with her.

She received specialist tuition weekly, differentiated worksheets and notes in class, and regular one-to-one discussion opportunities with her physics teacher.

While this took place in an independent setting, meaning access to funding and resources was less problematic, the engagement levels of her parents and the positive relationships between all stakeholders in Niamh's education meant that assessment and support led to appropriate provision. This underpinned Niamh's subsequent academic successes.

Building a working relationship with your child's school

Both parents and schools want the best for young people in our care. We want to support them to be their best selves, be ready to engage with the world independently and ultimately to be happy. In the ideal world, we are on the same team, working to support our children and young people. Many parents view schools as key in development of young people's self-esteem as well as providing academic input.

Positive, productive relationships are central to supporting young people. Where relationships are cordial and professional, young people benefit from support and provision that encompasses information from those that know them best and love them, as well as those with pedagogical knowledge, and access to the resources and systems within their setting.

When relationships break down, effective provision is risked as communication often falters and young people may disengage from support.

In this section, I suggest how to maintain constructive

relationships with your child's setting as well as signposting what you can do if relationships break down. I also present a case study where relationships majorly impacted on a student's and his parents' experiences of education.

CASE STUDY TWO – JONNY

Jonny was a low-attaining, Year 9 student. His Statement of Educational Need (the predecessor to an EHCP) was for his severe dyslexia. His journey to secondary school had been coloured by negative experiences at his primary school and he had very low self-esteem.

His parents felt that his primary school had caused his low confidence by not supporting him appropriately. He had made little progress and, while an eager learner, he found engaging with tasks at school very difficult. His parents felt unheard at school, despite calling meetings and raising their concerns during his time there. Even though Jonny had a Statement of Educational Need, his parents felt that the school was not meeting his needs.

After numerous meetings, informal and formal complaints at the school, relationships had broken down such that that Jonny's parents decided they would pursue a placement in specialist provision for Jonny. They engaged legal counsel as far as tribunal. However, the tribunal was unsuccessful, and Jonny remained in mainstream education.

His experiences of secondary education were much more positive. Prior to starting secondary school, the SEND team had contacted the family and described the support they would implement for Jonny when he started at the school. They then maintained contact throughout Key Stage 3.

The family felt that their concerns were heard and acted on, leading to a more positive experience of education for Jonny and the chance for him to pursue his interests at school, rebuilding his self-confidence and esteem.

Best ways to work with your child's school

Central to successful outcomes for your child are the relationships between those working with and supporting them through their education. Positive relationships with schools are fostered when schools communicate effectively with their community and seek their views regularly.

The key questions to be asked of your child's setting are outlined above and schools should address them regularly through termly (at least) reviews of your child's provision. The review process should incorporate your views and address any concerns you have with provision.

Staff working with your child should include your child in developing targets and outcomes which are then incorporated into their learning. Regular meetings with class teachers should take place; at least termly via meetings, parents' evenings, telephone consultations or other real-time interaction where possible. If meeting is not possible, written feedback should be given to parents and those supporting the child should be able to respond to concerns.

In reality, it is likely that your child's class teacher or form tutor will have contact with you more regularly than this as they are your main point of contact regarding most, if not all school matters. Form tutors and class teachers should support their tutees pastorally and may not actually teach their tutees. They aim to get to know your child and act as their advocate in school, where necessary. They should take time to get to know you, and work with you as a family so that you can collaboratively support your children.

Where this works, young people's needs may be met effectively, and concerns addressed in liaison with the school SENCO. However, where provision breaks down between you and your child's setting, negotiating provision adequately can be problematic.

Rocky relationships and what to do

Where relationships become fraught, it is often because parents feel that their child's needs are not being met or that they are not taken seriously. If you are concerned about your child's progress or provision, you don't have to leave discussions of it until the next scheduled meeting with teachers. Instead, contact them and organise a time to discuss your concerns so that they can be addressed before they escalate.

Preferably, write an email or letter to the school detailing your concerns before the meeting so that they know what you are worried about and have time to investigate and be ready to discuss ways forward with you at the meeting. If you have voiced your concerns in advance, teachers can better prepare. You will also be more confident as you have set the meeting agenda. Subsequently, any meeting or discussion will run smoothly, and issues will be ironed out.

If initial discussions and meetings are unfruitful, you can pursue more formal routes. The British Dyslexia Association Helpline may be able to provide guidance and general advice, or your local Dyslexia Association may be able to give you more area-specific guidance.

If, for example, the school refuses to apply for assessment for an EHCP, as a parent you have the right to do so, and the school must comply with any request for information. For more information on applying for an EHCP, visit the British Dyslexia Association website.[1]

Where you are dissatisfied with the support provided by the school and they are not forthcoming, you have the right to complain about that provision. Each school has a formal complaints procedure. If you wish to escalate your complaint further, local independent advice services are in place and will support you, providing guidance specific to your local area. There are also various advocacy services, both payable and free at point of use, which may be able to support you and your child should legal proceedings ensue.

♞ Key takeaways

- Your child's school should take steps if your child has indicators of dyslexia.

- Don't be afraid to ask questions about support for dyslexia.

- Maintain regular contact with the relevant staff.

- Be clear what you would like to happen and share this information ahead of meetings.

- If the relationship with your child's school breaks down, don't panic, there are options.

---

1 www.bdadyslexia.org.uk.

Further reading and resources

Policy and practice

Department for Education (DfE) (2014) 'Special educational needs and disabilities: A guide for parents and carers.' Accessed on March 2, 2021 at https://www.gov.uk/government/publications/send-guide-for-parents-and-carers.

Department for Education (DfE) (2014) 'The young person's guide to the Children and Families Act 2014.' Accessed on March 2, 2021 at https://assets.publishing.service.gov.uk/government/uploads/system/uploads/attachment_data/file/359681/Young_Person_s_Guide_to_the_Children_and_Families_Act.pdf.

Department for Education (DfE) (2020) 'Ask, Listen, Do: A guide to making conversations count for all families.' Accessed on March 2, 2021 at https://www.sendgateway.org.uk/resources/ask-listen-do-guide-making-conversations-count-all-families.

Education, Health and Care Plans (EHCP)

Council for Disabled Children (2014) 'The SEND Reforms: A Guide to Education Health and Care Plans.' Accessed on March 2, 2021 at https://issuu.com/councilfordisabledchildren/docs/send_reforms_guide_to_ehc_plans_201.

Council for Disabled Children (2014) 'Education, Health and Care Plans.' Accessed on March 2, 2021 at https://councilfordisabled-children.org.uk/sites/default/files/uploads/documents/import/a4l-letehcfinal3.pdf.

Contacts

UK Government (n.d.) 'Children with special educational needs and disabilities (SEND).' Accessed on March 2, 2021 at https://www.gov.uk/children-with-special-educational-needs/special-educational-needs-support.

Council for Disabled Children (n.d.) 'Find your local IAS Service.' Accessed on March 2, 2021 at https://councilfordisabledchildren. org.uk/information-advice-and-support-services-network/find-your-local-ias-service.

— CHAPTER 10 —

Supporting Your Child's Emotional Development

PENNIE ASTON

Summary

◇ Why a dyslexic child is more vulnerable to low self-esteem and how to rebuild it.

◇ Importance of general wellbeing to you and your dyslexic child.

◇ Dyslexia and constant anxiety, and how to manage it.

◇ Why you should focus on strengths, and the many strengths dyslexia can bring to focus on.

◇ The importance of being kind and listening to yourself and your dyslexic child.

How do we emotionally support our dyslexic child? It's the question we all ask ourselves, usually when things are falling apart and we are the ones who are desperate for support. This chapter is all about putting things in place before this happens, and understanding the 'why?' so we can preempt negative fallout, both for ourselves and our children.

Do dyslexic children have a harder time containing their emotions? I believe they do, for a number of reasons.

First, they are in the minority and they often sense their so-called difference, but can't put words to it. They just feel unlike their peers. As adults we can be fairly logical about a dyslexia assessment, but for a child it can often mean that they feel odd and out of step.

Second, when you feel odd and out of step, you will pretty much do anything to be like everyone else in the hope that then things will be 'normal'. I actually have no idea what 'normal' feels like, but it does seem to be a quest that many dyslexic people have. When you are looking for something but don't exactly know what it is, how will you recognise it? That is the emotional dilemma.

We are all wonderfully, beautifully unique, but the dyslexic child can have real problems with individuation – as an example, not knowing if they will pass or fail a test, depending on how the test is given. Then, not being able to own their successes or cope with their failures because they are emotionally preparing themselves for the worst all the time. At this point, they have reached despair, which impacts profoundly on self-esteem.

In order to build up their self-esteem, we have to under-stand exactly what it is and where it comes from.

Self-esteem

We all need self-esteem in order to cope with the world. But what exactly is it and where do we get it from?

Put simply, it's about feeling loved and competent. It's about being able to manage our emotions and being able to control and express ourselves in acceptable ways. When we can do that, we feel better about ourselves and in control of our environment. Feeling calm and accepted helps us to achieve our goals and leads to happier lives.

Let's be honest though – how many dyslexic people, child or adult, feel that they have been accepted and appreciated just as they are? How many of us manage all of this, all of the time?

In many ways, developing and maintaining self-esteem is a continuous quest – a learning path from the moment we are born. Dyslexic people often have a harder job of this because of their life experiences, especially through the education system.

Why is self-esteem so important?

Self-esteem is important because feeling good about who we are enables us to learn more effectively. It helps us to cope with life's stresses and strains and inspires us to create a better future for ourselves.

There's a general recognition that self-esteem is a primary factor in the building and maintenance of social and emotional wellbeing. Someone who has a healthy level of self-esteem is more likely to achieve at their full potential and form successful relationships than a person who suffers from acute feelings of lack of self-worth. In other words, it is what makes the world go round and we cannot underestimate its importance in all areas of our dyslexic lives. Without it, we can fall into the well of low self-esteem.

What is low self-esteem?

Because of these life experiences, some dyslexic children grow up placing little value on their abilities and often deny their successes. They find it difficult to set goals and to problem solve.

The end result is that many give up trying and consequently perform well below their academic and social capabilities. These self-limiting beliefs become self-fulfilling prophecies and this is what we mean by having low self-esteem. People can tell your child over and over how well they've done, but they will probably believe the one person who says they need to do better.

This is particularly prevalent when your child is dyslexic and their abilities are judged on a limited number of attributes and rarely on their strengths. They focus unrelentingly on what they find challenging, what others seem to find easy, and often categorise themselves as thick, stupid and useless.

What can we do to build self-esteem?

The best way to start is to be the very best role model you are capable of being to your child. If you have unresolved issues around your own or their dyslexia, this is the time to address them. We can all be angry about an education system that may be unsupportive, but are we as parents truly accepting of our dyslexic child? If not, how can we expect the child to be truly accepting of themselves?

We need to actually demonstrate positive behaviours so our children can learn from us. We can do this by talking. Help your child to talk about their problems and feelings.

This helps them to start being familiar with how they react in given situations and what the options might be.

A word of warning here – no 'fixing'! They don't need fixing. They need to really know themselves – what they are good at and what can be a challenge. Often the dyslexic child is trying so hard to be like everyone else to fit in that they lose sight of who they actually are – as do we as adults.

Next, we need to help them build some coping skills. Work with your child to learn skills to problem solve. Challenge any negative thinking with an enquiry. What can we do about a given situation? What are the options? Nothing is more fearful than feeling powerless and in this way we help our children to realise their strengths, even if they are not the ones that get perfect grades in tests.

Promoting general wellbeing

Meanwhile, we must look after their wellbeing. Are we promoting their healthy eating and physical activity? Are we promoting our own? Children model what they see, so this is a brilliant time to start doing things with them. This helps to bond our relationship with them, providing intimacy and connection. Exercise is a great tool to boost mood and reduce stress and anxiety.

This is all self-care and we need to promote that with our child so that they have time and space to look after themselves. Involve yourself in their hobbies. Do the activity with them. Be the bystander rooting for them.

This helps your child to develop autonomy. Allow them to make their own decisions. This, in turn, helps them to build resilience so they are able to bounce back when the world knocks them down, knowing they will survive and thrive and be back to fight another day.

If all these things are in place, your child will be better placed to build positive relationships. Relationships are a vital part of growing emotionally; they allow us to feel connected to and respected by others, but first and foremost we need to connect to and respect ourselves.

Relaxation is something we think we know how to do, but we may fail to appreciate the benefits it can bring. In our society, we are rushing from one thing to another often with little time or space to reflect or wind down. Teach your child some relaxation skills, like deep breathing. Listen to a short meditation recording together. Be seen doing it yourself so your child will be intrigued and want to try it themselves.

Promote play and creativity with your child. Things may be tough at school and play can calm a ruffled nervous system down. Give them time to explore things, enquire about things, try things without judgement or fear of 'getting it wrong'.

Finally, how are your sleep habits? Regular bedtime? A 'no screens in the bedroom' family rule? Do you have wind down time half an hour before sleep time to prompt the brain to start developing melatonin (which encourages sleep)? If you answer 'yes' to all these questions, then great. If not, perhaps this can be a project for everyone, because it certainly will help.

You may be thinking by now, 'That's all well and good but how do I do all these things?' I have no easy answers, other than to say the more you do them, the easier they get. The more rehearsal you do, the easier it is to contend with difficult situations when they arise. And as we know, difficult situations do arise for the dyslexic child all the time. When they do we are faced with their anxiety and ours, often at a time when we are least able to call on any reserves. So, please, get practising.

Here's a short reminder list:

◇ be a role model

◇ talk to your child

◇ develop their coping skills

◇ promote wellbeing

◇ encourage autonomy

◇ support relationships

◇ relaxation

◇ play

◇ sleep.

Dealing with anxiety

Nothing in the world is perfect and even with the best-laid plans and support strategies, anxiety can strike us all.

The difficulty for the dyslexic child is that anxiety can be an ever-present feeling. They have learnt to be on guard, especially at school, every minute of every day, of every week of every month. You get the idea!

Many people have said to me, 'Everyone gets anxious.' Well, yes, they do, but it is often occasionally and for good reason. For the dyslexic child it can be all the time. Often, they will be able to hold it all in at school, but then the reserves break down at home. The child you have is unrecognisable to the child they see at school. As heart-breaking as this may be to you, know one thing. If your child falls apart when they get home, it is because they know they can. They know they are safe. Their nervous system can begin to start trying to even out. That emotional outburst is often the only way the child knows how to communicate their distress.

If all the strategies mentioned above to deal with self-esteem are in place, then we have a better chance of bringing things onto an even keel and encouraging clear communication. If not, we need to understand a little more about anxiety and why it happens.

Anxiety is actually our friend. It's a survival technique from our Neanderthal past. The person who was alert and on guard was the one who survived to pass on their DNA. Great if you are in the Stone Age. Not so great when you live in the 21st century.

Our world goes at such a fast pace that it is hard to keep up as an adult (which is why we too need to put our self-esteem strategies into effect). Imagine what it is like for a child. Especially one that is being tested and evaluated, scored and judged and is utterly powerless.

The brain starts deciding that there are lots of things to be wary of. That wonderful dyslexic brain that can hold loads of ideas all at the same time and make amazing connections is the same brain that can be thinking of everything that might possibly go wrong at any given point. That's not a brain that can commit itself to be able to learn. In fact, the survival mechanism triggers the brain to zip into fight or flight mode. That mode is deep in our reptilian brain and, for reasons of survival, it disconnects from the 'thinking' brain. How can a child be expected to learn when their nervous system is primed for survival?

For all these reasons, we need to be able to identify when

anxiety or anxious processes are occurring. Here's a list to help you recognise anxiety in yourself and your child:

- memory issues
- overthinking
- avoidance
- sweating
- stomach issues
- panic attacks
- needing reassurance
- procrastination
- trouble breathing
- constant worrying
- trouble concentrating
- lack of patience
- headaches
- rapid heartbeat
- insomnia.

This is not a nice list of symptoms to experience and it is even less nice when you are watching your child go through it. This is why it is so important to perfect those self-esteem approaches in the first place so you have strategies to call on that are familiar and have become second nature.

But if you haven't, what do you do? The following is a list that I personally use and have found very helpful with clients.

What to tell myself (or my child) when I'm feeling anxious:

- This feeling won't last forever.

- Thoughts and emotions aren't facts.

- I can feel anxious and still handle this.

- My bravery is stronger than my fear.

- I am safe right now.

- Anxiety is reminding me to slow down my breathing.

- I've survived other tough times before, and I will be resilient this time too.

- This feeling is a normal reaction. I will use my coping tools to respond with thoughtfulness and self-compassion.

- I don't have to figure this all out right now. I will trust the process.

- Thank you, anxiety, for always trying to look out for me, but it's okay now, I've got this.

- Oh hello! There's that thought again – and it is just a thought.

Copy this list out and read through it out loud when things get tough.

Sometimes it helps to ask your child what sort of animal their anxiety might be. This may sound a bit strange but ask yourself how easily you could answer the question, 'What's wrong?' Often there is so much going on that the child is completely overwhelmed and unable to verbalise their worries. But 'bear' or 'spider' or even 'monster' gets it out of their brain and into the conversation. You could also ask what animal they need to be to deal with their anxiety. What fears do they have? You can then role-play. Be creative and have fun with it. Model 'doing' something, not being 'victim' to it.

Focusing on strengths

One way of supporting the development of self-esteem and helping to minimise anxiety is to focus on strengths.

We are all good at something. Sadly, the dyslexic child often gets to believe that there is nothing they can get right. As their parent, it is your job and privilege to escort your youngster through the trials and tribulations of growing up while taking the rough edge off their frustration. The day-to-day demands of growing up as a dyslexic person in a predominantly linear world can take its toll – both on you and your child.

Children will always do well if they can. They do poorly when life demands skills that they are lacking. That is the fault of the way they are being taught, not a deficit in the child.

What we can do is figure out what their strengths are. What doesn't work for them? What does work for them? What do they love? The following list is one that I worked on with 11-year-old Ben. Ben was beginning to find things really hard and was getting extremely anxious. This was impacting on every area of his life.

My name is Ben. I am 11 years old.

My strengths are:

- visual learner

- empathetic and compassionate

- good friend

- resourceful

- observant – I notice things most others don't

- inventiveness

- perseverance

- resilience.

(NB: these are not things you can easily evaluate but they make you a pretty awesome human being.)

What doesn't work for me:

- punishment

- power struggling

- taking away physical outlets

- pressure to perform

- shaming

- passive aggression

- lecturing

- self-starting.

(You may look at this list and note how many of these things wind you up as well.)

What does work for me:

- trust that I am trying

- building a relationship and trust

- loud, fun and engaging lessons

- patience

- proactive strategies

- allowing lots of breaks to move around

- discreet, private clues to redirect

- positive reinforcement and feedback

- oral and visual directions combined.

What I love:

- any animal

- playing football with my friends

- playing jokes on my Dad

- chocolate.

This gives us a much more all-round sense of Ben. Stuff is going on that he is finding difficult. He feels that he can't get anything right. But when we work together, he can see that there is a lot of good in the things he does. You can do the lists as many times as you like and remember, *praise* is what dyslexic children thrive on.

Refer back to the list, 'What to tell myself (or my child) when I'm feeling anxious'. Use it to prompt conversation to fill in the topic headings. If your child finds it hard to think of personal strengths, here is a list that may prompt them to think differently (which is everything we are working towards):

- ◇ innovative and imaginative thinker

- ◇ good visualisation and spatial skills

- ◇ often creative – good sense of colour and texture, may excel at art, design and photography

- ◇ thinks in pictures, which is quicker and more multi-directional than thinking in words

- ◇ good verbally

- ◇ can be very humorous

- ◇ may be good at the performing arts

- ◇ holistic – sees the whole picture

- ◇ can multitask

- ◇ intuitive problem solver

- ◇ often hard working and tenacious

- ◇ high emotional intelligence, empathetic

- ◇ good interpersonal skills

- ◇ valuable and supportive team member

- ◇ entrepreneurial

- ◇ often very charming

- ◇ friendly and outgoing, may be entertaining and amusing

- ◇ good verbally, may be powerful speakers

- ◇ passionate about subjects or causes

- ◇ lateral thinkers

- ◇ innovative

- ◇ creative

- ◇ doggedly determined.

Did that surprise you? Do you recognise any of them? Most information about dyslexia tends to focus on the bad stuff but there's a lot of good about it and that's what we need to focus on with our children.

Have a think about the following points.

Seeing the bigger picture

People with dyslexia often see things more holistically. They miss the trees, but see the forest.

Finding the odd one out

People with dyslexia excel at global visual processing and the detection of impossible figures. Scientist Christopher Tonkin, who has dyslexia, described his unusual sensitivity to 'things out of place' (Schneps 2014). Scientists in his line of work must make sense of enormous quantities of visual data and accurately find black hole anomalies.

There are so many people with dyslexia in the field of astrophysics that it prompted research at the Harvard-Smithsonian Center for Astrophysics. Findings confirmed that those with dyslexia are better at identifying and memorising complex images (Schneps 2014).

Improved pattern recognition

People with dyslexia have the ability to see how things connect to form complex systems and to identify similarities among multiple things. Such strengths are likely to be of particular significance for fields like science and mathematics, where visual representations are key.

Good spatial knowledge

Many people with dyslexia demonstrate better skills at manipulating 3D objects in their mind. Many of the world's top architects and fashion designers have dyslexia.

Picture thinkers

People with dyslexia tend to think in pictures rather than words. Research at the University of California has demonstrated children who have dyslexia also have enhanced picture recognition memory (Hedenius *et al.* 2013).

Nineteenth-century French sculptor Auguste Rodin could stare at paintings in museums by day and paint them from memory at night. His dyslexia meant he could barely read or write by the age of 14, with his reading skills developing much later.

Sharper peripheral vision

People with dyslexia have better peripheral vision than most, meaning they can quickly take in a whole scene.

Although it can be hard to focus in on individual words, dyslexia seems to make it easier to see outer edges. James Howard Jr, a professor of psychology at the Catholic University of America, described in the journal *Neuropsychologia* an experiment in which participants were asked to pick out the letter T from a sea of letter L's floating on a computer screen (Howard *et al.* 2006). Those with dyslexia identified the letter more quickly.

Business entrepreneurs

Did you know that one in three American entrepreneurs have dyslexia (see Logan 2009)?

Entrepreneurs like Thomas Edison, Henry Ford, Steve Jobs, Bill Gates and Charles Schwab all are/were dyslexic people, as is our own Richard Branson. Perhaps better strategic and creative thinking could provide a real business advantage.

Highly creative

Many of the world's most creative actors have dyslexia, such as Johnny Depp, Keira Knightley and Orlando Bloom.

The artist Pablo Picasso was described by his teachers as 'having difficulty differentiating the orientation of letters'. Picasso painted his subjects as he saw them – sometimes out of order, backwards or upside down. His paintings demonstrated the power of his imagination, which was perhaps linked to his inability to see written words properly.

Richard Rogers, the British architect, has created countless beautiful buildings; he is best known for his work on the Pompidou Centre in Paris, the Lloyd's building and Millennium Dome in London, the Senedd in Cardiff, and the European Court of Human Rights building in Strasbourg. Rogers did not excel academically, which made him believe that he was 'stupid' because he couldn't read or memorise his school work and as a consequence he stated that he 'became very depressed'.[1] He wasn't able to read until the age of 11 and it was not until after he had his first child that he realised that he was dyslexic.

Thinking outside the box – problem solving

Dyslexic people are well known for having sudden leaps of insight that solve problems with an unorthodox approach. This is an intuitive approach to problem solving that can seem like daydreaming. Staring out of the window is how dyslexia works, letting the brain slide into neutral and ease itself around a problem to let connections assemble.

Dyslexic strengths are subtle and powerful, and not easy to define. When much of what a child has experienced is a feeling of not quite doing things right and not knowing what to do to make it right, they will need reassurance and proof that this will not be forever and their time will come. You have to believe it too.

---

1   https://www.nessy.com/us/parents/dyslexia-information/9-strengths-dyslexia.

In that vein let's have a look at what those standardised tests can't measure.

- Affection
- Character
- Common sense
- Compassion
- Confidence
- Courage
- Creativity
- Determination
- Diligence
- Discernment
- Effort
- Empathy
- Faith
- Faithfulness
- Flexibility
- Fortitude
- Friendliness
- Generosity
- Gentleness
- Grit
- Helpfulness
- Honesty
- Ingenuity
- Intelligence
- Intuition
- Joy
- Kindness
- Life skills
- Love
- Love of learning
- Loyalty
- Manners
- Morals
- Motivation
- Passion
- Peacefulness
- Perseverance
- Personality
- Perspective
- Physical fitness

- Resilience
- Rhythm
- Self-control
- Self-esteem
- Sense of humour
- Spirituality
- Strength
- Thoroughness
- Wit
- Work ethic

How many of these qualities does your child possess? Which ones would they like to work towards? As they move towards a more positive and well-rounded sense of who they are, we as their guides and guardians can help direct them to understand what they can and what they can't control.

Learning what you can and what you can't control

Once there is a better sense of the positive qualities your child holds, another good strategy for focusing on strengths, reducing anxiety and developing self-esteem is to know what you can and can't control.

Below is the work of 13-year-old Holly who was feeling that she didn't fit in and believed she was finding things so much harder than most of her peer group. We worked on examining what was going on in her life which, to her, felt overwhelming. We then split the list into two columns.

I can control	I can't control
Doing my homework	Someone else's decision
Respecting property	Death
Being kind	Who likes me
Being accountable	How others treat me
Studying for tests	Others taking care of
The friends I choose to have	themselves
My decisions	Others being kind
Forgiving	Who loves me
How I respond to challenges	My height
Trying again	My skin colour
How I spend my free time	Past mistakes
Doing my chores	Others being honest
Being honest	If someone else keeps trying
Taking care of myself	Weather
Working hard	Others forgiving me
Asking for help	Others asking for help
How I respond to others	Others apologising to me
Apologising	

During the process (which took a fair bit of time and conversation), she was able to see that she had lots of strengths that she was ignoring. She was also getting a sense of whether what she was feeling was because of other people's behaviours or because of how she was viewing herself. To get a sense of control, a sense of having some autonomy, the following is useful to remind your child:

I can't control anyone else, but I can control:

◇ my thoughts

◇ my words

◇ my choices

◇ my actions

- ◇ my reactions

- ◇ my future.

Whatever situation they are in, we know it won't last forever. But they do not have the life experience as yet to believe it. Refer back to the 'what to tell myself (or my child) when I'm feeling anxious' list and read it out loud with your child. The reading out loud helps to embed the words, allows them to 'feel all the feelings' safely and strengthen their self-esteem. Refer back to the list of strengths they have and work through them again.

Sometimes, though, the behaviour becomes too much and parents are driven to distraction. It's okay. You are only human. It's worth keeping in mind that behaviours that we find intolerable are often the only way the child knows how (as yet) to express their distress.

Parenting guidelines

What we've been looking at is how we can raise self-esteem and reduce the felt anxiety of our dyslexic children. Equally important in emotionally supporting our child is looking after ourselves and placing limits or boundaries on behaviour (theirs and ours). This is valuable to your child as they mirror behaviour that they are exposed to and are quick to pick up on any hypocrisy – this is especially true of the super-sensitive, intuitive dyslexic child that notices every mannerism, micro-expression, tone of voice and gesture.

In the first place, be kind to yourself!

I have found the work of Kristin Neff to be very valuable.[2] In essence, she promotes self-compassion and believes it is that value that equals a happy life. Parents of dyslexic children can be very hard on themselves especially when they don't know what to do to support their child when they see they are anguished. In essence, the following are excellent principles to follow:

⬧ **Self-kindness**: We are as caring toward ourselves as we are toward others.

⬧ **Recognising our common humanity**: Moments of connection with others and the shared human experience.

⬧ **Mindfulness**: Being open to the reality of the present moment. Acknowledging our suffering without exaggerating it.

I would add a fourth which I call The Golden Rule. Treat others as you would like (or would have liked) to be treated yourself. Keep that in mind as we journey through the minefield of what to do as a parent of a dyslexic child.

As well as being kind to ourselves we also have a duty of care to sort out our own stuff and heal our own wounds. If you are dyslexic yourself and discover you have a dyslexic child, it can kick up all kinds of emotional baggage left over from your own unresolved experiences. If so, do all the strategies we've already covered for yourself before you work with your child. It's also worth us taking a look at how we are interpreting behaviour. Have a think about the following:

---

2   https://self-compassion.org.

When a child...	They could be feeling...
whines...	powerless, unable to cope, need to cry.
is bossy or controlling...	concerned they won't get their needs met.
is taunting or competitive...	undervalued for who they are and may need more connection.
won't listen...	that their needs are unacknowledged.
is rebellious...	powerless and incompetent.
is disrespectful...	a lack of connectedness with you.
is hurtful...	hurt.

Always remind yourself to look for what's hiding behind the 'misbehaviours'. This may be the only vocabulary your child knows to make you aware of how they are feeling.

Let's have a look now at how you react. When faced with difficult and challenging behaviour, what is your response? Keep in mind that your words matter and giving your child boundaries will help them to develop emotional intelligence and self-regulation. Have a look at the following alternatives that may help:

Instead of...	Try...
Be quiet...	Can you use a softer voice?
What a mess!...	It looks like you had fun! How can we clean up?
Do you need help?...	I'm here to help if you need me.
I explained how to do this yesterday...	Maybe I can show you another way.
Do I need to separate you?...	Could you use a break?
Stop crying...	It's okay to cry.
Do you have any questions?...	What questions do you have?
You're okay...	How are you feeling?
not that hard...	You can do hard things.
don't talk like that...	Please use kind words.

As you get more used to phrasing clean, clear, language with boundaries it opens up options for your child to make choices. Refer back here to 'Learning what you can and what you can't control'.

Another approach that can help is 'time-ins'. In a time-in, a child who is having a hard time is invited to sit with us for comfort and calming. During this time we help the child to express their feelings and point of view, listening to and empathising with them. This co-regulation calms their frazzled nervous system. When the child is calm, we then explain why the behaviour is not okay and help the child problem solve the situation. We may discuss alternative ways of addressing the situation in an age-appropriate way and get their input and ideas. A time-in will always involve a two-way conversation where we actively listen to what the child is saying and respect the child's perspective and feelings.

Time-ins help children to learn to self-regulate, provide opportunities for them to explain their needs, help them understand the effect their choices have on others, and offer problem solving opportunities for current and future situations. Time-ins also support emotional intelligence. During a time-in:

◇ children feel that their needs are being considered

◇ we strengthen the connection between us and the child

◇ children are given time to identify and process feelings

◇ we avoid power struggles and prevent escalation of force, as both of us co-regulate

◇ children don't feel isolated, scared or shamed

- ◇ children participate in finding solutions, which will help should a similar situation arise in the future

- ◇ children learn through role modelling and conversation how to problem solve calmly, respectfully and non-violently.

As you will notice, time-ins nicely combine all the strategies we have already covered. Instead of using a consequence like 'time-out', which excludes the child, try some of the following:

Put in a boundary...	I won't let you hit; let's sit here together while we keep playing.
Connect...	I can see you are getting really frustrated. How can I help?
Model regulation...	I can see you're feeling really mad, let's stomp! Let's get all that energy out through our feet!
Collaborate and teach...	Once the emotion has settled, collaboratively discuss new ways of managing big emotions.

Apologies

It's worth spending a little time thinking about what an apology actually is and is not. Adults seem to find it particularly difficult to admit to a child that they got things wrong and yet it is one of the most powerful things to model – that we can be wrong, admit to it and move on.

An apology is not...	An apology is...
I'm sorry you feel that way...	I'm sorry I hurt you.
That was not my intention...	I will be more mindful of this in future.
Maybe you're upset because this is one of your triggers...	I know you are sensitive about this. I messed up.
You are making a big deal out of nothing...	I'm sorry. Can you help me understand why this hurts?

Active listening

Lastly, I can recommend the use of active listening. Dyslexic people can be very tuned in to body language, tone of voice, micro-expressions and authenticity. Often, they can't explain in words what they feel – they 'just know'. This is to do with their higher level, global thinking skills. However, they often don't come with an experience of being listened to as their inward dialogue and visual imagination can create delays in processing. Dyslexic people often think in pictures, which they then have to 'translate' into words. The time it takes to do this can be excessive with lots of stops and starts.

REMEMBER

◇ Take the time to really listen to your child.

◇ Listen to understand – not to reply.

◇ Note what they said and how you felt about it.

◇ Clarify that you have heard them correctly.

◇ Give them time and space to think, process and reply.

Conclusion

Now we are at the end of this short chapter but at the beginning of developing skills to emotionally support your dyslexic child. We are not seeking to make everything all okay and fix things. We are endeavouring to develop skills that build resilience, emotional intelligence, self-knowledge, trust in self and others and a sense of knowing you can survive difficult situations

We've done this by looking at what self-esteem is, how you can build it and how to cope with anxiety, focusing on strengths and some parenting guidelines. All it needs now is practice.

Remember as you work with your child that things take time to embed and be thoroughly understood. It takes time to understand the benefits, subtle as they can be. It's very easy to give up when things become a bit difficult. I would encourage you to keep on keeping on. You are building strong foundations for a positive, emotionally healthy relationship with your child that will last a lifetime.

🏵 Key takeaways

- Don't seek to make everything all okay and fix things. Endeavour to support your child to develop the skills that build resilience, emotional intelligence, self-knowledge, trust in self and others, and a sense of knowing they can survive difficult situations.

- Practise building self-esteem, coping with anxiety, focusing on strengths and general parenting guidelines.

- It takes time to understand and see the benefits your

support has on your dyslexic child's emotional development, and the changes can be subtle.

- Don't give up when things become a bit difficult. Keep on
keeping on.

- The strategies discussed in this chapter will build strong
foundations for a positive and emotionally healthy
relationship with your child that will last a lifetime.

References

Hedenius, M., Ullman, M.T., Alm, P., Jennische, M. & Persson, J.
(2013) 'Enhanced recognition memory after incidental encoding
in children with developmental dyslexia.' *PloS ONE 8*, 5, e63998.
https://journals.plos.org/plosone/article?id=10.1371/journal.
pone.0063998.
Howard, J.H., Jr., Howard, D.V., Japikse, K.A. & Eden, G.F. (2006)
'Dyslexics are impaired on implicit higher-order sequence learning,
but not on spatial context learning.' *Neuropsychologia 44*, 1131–
1144.
Logan, J. (2009) 'Dyslexic entrepreneurs: The incidence; their coping
strategies and their business skills.' *Dyslexia 15*, 4, 328–346.
Schneps, M.H. (2014) 'The advantages of dyslexia.' *Scientific
American*, August 19. Accessed on January 21, 2021 at https://
www.scientificamerican.com/article/the-advantages-of-dyslexia.

Further reading and resources

Haines, S. (2018) *Anxiety Is Really Strange*. London: Singing Dragon.
Johnstone, M. (2015) *The Little Book of Resilience: How to Bounce
Back from Adversity and Lead a Fulfilling Life*. London: Robinson.
Portmann, R. (2008) *The 50 Best Games for Building Self-Esteem*.
Buckingham: Hinton House.

'Wheel of Emotions', developed by psychologist Robert Plutchik, is a brightly coloured visual prompt for working with your child. Many versions are available online, e.g. https://thesensorytoolbox.com/plutchiks-wheel-of-emotions.

Conclusion

Well done, you have made it through the handbook. You might have read and re-read certain chapters as you try to understand what dyslexia is and whether your child might have dyslexia. You might have planned a way forward with the next steps decided upon. Chapters 1–5 are informative on the process involved in deciding on undertaking an assessment.

It is likely the journey will not be straightforward and you might experience highs and lows, ups and downs. Some of the downs will be the result of struggles your child may be having with, for example, reading. It is common to notice initial progress, but find that it slows as the curriculum increases in difficulty. At these challenging times, it is important to focus on self-esteem by offering lots of praise and encouragement. Focus on the young person's strengths in areas in which they feel they are successful. Help them to develop strategies for tasks they are finding difficult. The handbook is a practical guide for you to keep coming back to. The key features of Chapters 6–10 are the tips and strategies for skills which your child will continue to develop throughout their time in education. Collectively, they cover the individual steps made when learning to read. Chapters 7 and 8 focus on the organisational side of learning and how best to study. Remember to begin to develop these skills with your child from an early age, not just when they move up into Key Stage 4 (at age 14).

As your child develops independence as a learner, one of the key areas to explore is assistive technology. There is software for all different aspects of learning. Chapter 3 highlights how using software which alleviates reading or writing enables learners to understand text or to get their thoughts onto paper without writing. Assistive technology will be included as recommendations in any Diagnostic Assessment and Chapter 4 covers this. Chapter 6 explores in more depth a range of situations where you might use software for mind mapping, or phonic development or spelling and writing.

As we look forwards in the field of dyslexia research, assistive technology is an area which is growing exponentially. For children and young people with dyslexia, it offers them a range of tools which effectively level the playing field with their peers. It enables them to produce work which is reflective of their ability rather than their barriers. If we help our children to explore how best they learn and work, we are giving them the ability to work independently. This is the door to a successful future. With the right assistive technology, dyslexic children can and do thrive throughout life, especially if as parents and carers, you are able to empower them to identify the resources like assistive technology, that will support them, and the self-understanding to see their own strengths, which we have shown in this book to be so vital to their self-esteem and therefore wellbeing.

The ultimate journey for any child with dyslexia is to be able to step out into the world of work. Dyslexia is considered a disability under the definition in the Equality Act (2010).

This means the challenges which are experienced by people with dyslexia are recognised and reasonable adjustments can be made to enable them to work effectively. We can help our children by beginning to explore how they can be successful and what tools they will need at a young age. This is the importance of assistive technology and essentially the take home message of the handbook.

Contributors

Gillian Ashley is a qualified teacher and has had a career in teaching across primary, secondary, pupil referral unit (PRU) and university levels. Gillian oversaw whole school SEND in a variety of educational settings. Gillian specialised in dyslexia and qualified as a Dyslexia Specialist. She completed an MA in Additional Learning Needs. She then carried out research into prosody and reading comprehension as part of her Masters in Psychology. Gillian has led a Masters in Dyslexia and Dyscalculia at university level. She is currently the Chief Development Officer at The British Dyslexia Association.

Pennie Aston is the Founder and Director of GroOops Dyslexia Aware Counselling, an organisation that focuses exclusively on developing counselling and psycho-social programmes that address the emotional repercussions of dyslexia in particular and neurodiversity generally. She is dyslexic herself and has raised a neurodiverse family.

Katrina Cochrane is a Specialist Teacher and Assessor who has been working in the field of dyslexia for over 20 years. She has co-written two books on dyslexia as well as helped to write the BDA Level 7 course for Specialist Teachers/Assessors. She set up her company Positive Dyslexia, after leaving the BDA in 2016, where she was Head of Education and Policy. Katrina remains a member of the BDA Accreditation Board and is an Associate Trainer and Assessor for the BDA.

Adam Gordon is the SEND and Inclusion Manager at LGfL (www.lgfl.net). He is passionate about helping schools to improve inclusive practice and support learners with additional needs. As someone who has dyslexia, Adam has experienced his own challenges in education. As a teaching assistant, teacher, assistant headteacher and in his current role, Adam has always been passionate about engaging, relevant and accessible education for all, and he believes that technology has a powerful part to play in enabling this.

Dr Lindsay Peer CBE is one the UK's leading dyslexia experts with decades of expertise on working directly with young people with dyslexia and in academia. She is also the mother of children with dyslexia. She is a practitioner psychologist, international speaker, author and expert witness. In 2002, she was appointed CBE for services to education and dyslexia. She is a Patron of GroOops, a charity dedicated to creating an emotionally healthy, dyslexia aware world. In 2011, she was presented with an Outstanding Lifetime Academic Achievement Award by the British Dyslexia Association, where she previously held the posts of Education Director and Deputy CEO.

Dr Helen Ross is a researcher-practitioner whose research informs her work as a Specialist Assessor, SEN teacher and education consultant. She has worked with local government, the British Dyslexia Association, and central government inter alia to evaluate programmes, provide evidence-based policy recommendations and undertake targeted research projects. Helen is also Chair of the Wiltshire Dyslexia Association.

Index